"Glandion Carney's *The Way of Grace* is a gift from the heart of one of the very best spiritual directors I have ever known. For some, receiving the dreaded diagnosis of Parkinson's would be a death knell, but for my friend Glandion, it became the occasion to ring a different bell, and to mine his own soul for lessons of grace. This is a book for anyone wrestling with issues of theodicy."

Gary W. Moon, executive director of the Dallas Willard Center, Westmont College, and author of *Apprenticeship with Jesus*

"I love this book! It captures the prayerful and compassionate heart of Glandion Carney, a man I was privileged to work alongside in pastoral ministry. Beautifully written, it also reflects the heart of the coauthor, Marjean Brooks—a beautiful woman of deep faith and prayer, graced with the Spirit of God as a writer, teacher, mentor and friend. I highly recommend *The Way of Grace* to anyone who desires to see beyond the pain to the goodness, complexity and yet the simplicity of the grace of God. Every chapter points to Jesus, full of grace and truth."

Karen Mahler, assistant pastor of pastoral care, St. Peter's Anglican Church, Birmingham, Alabama

"Glandion Carney and Marjean Brooks have written a riveting and soul-piercing book describing his experiences in learning to live with Parkinson's. His inspiring understanding about the amazing grace of God within the deserts of life is applicable to everyone on the journey of faith. We can all learn from reading his story, and will come away knowing how to recognize and receive God's grace in our own hard places."

Foley Beach, bishop, Anglican Diocese of the South

"*The Way of Grace* shatters the . . . belief that God's grace appears in forms of prosperity, good fortune, acclaim, the job we wanted or the perfect children. But it reassembles the reality of a grace experienced in unexpected, unsought afflictions and circumstances.... A remarkable book of a remarkable God and a man humbled and gifted by brokenness. A hope for all who suffer, who know others who suffer and for all who want to embrace life in the midst of debilitation and dying. For is that not the lot of all who inhabit this broken world?"

Jane Rubietta, speaker and author of *Finding Life: From Eden to Gethsemane*

"Glandion Carney walks the path that Jesus walked. He follows him with a cheerful heart, no matter how hard the way. Stones confront us: stern and rugged terrain. But God's grace empowers us. Glandion's charm and steadfast love of the Savior warm and enlighten us in these pages. He relates with simplicity a life lived in trust, in spite of suffering, weakness, aging or illness. Glandion's wisdom shows us a Lord who guards our every step on the toughest mountain path."

Emilie Griffin, author of *Souls in Full Sail* and *Green Leaves for Later Years*

"Like Glandion in person, Glandion in book form is always the 'real deal.' Anyone facing a seeming debilitating transition or walking alongside that person needs Glandion at their side, telling them both the truths and stories contained in this marvelous book."

Jan Johnson, author of *Abundant Simplicity* and *Renovation of the Heart in Daily Practice*

THE
WAY
OF
GRACE

FINDING GOD ON THE
PATH OF SURRENDER

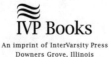

GLANDION CARNEY
with MARJEAN BROOKS

Foreword by RICHARD J. FOSTER

IVP Books

An imprint of InterVarsity Press
Downers Grove, Illinois

InterVarsity Press
P.O. Box 1400, Downers Grove, IL 60515-1426
World Wide Web: www.ivpress.com
Email: email@ivpress.com

*InterVarsity Press® is the book-publishing division of InterVarsity Christian Fellowship/USA®, a
movement of students and faculty active on campus at hundreds of universities, colleges and schools of
nursing in the United States of America, and a member movement of the International Fellowship of
Evangelical Students. For information about local and regional activities, write Public Relations
Dept., InterVarsity Christian Fellowship/USA, 6400 Schroeder Rd., P.O. Box 7895, Madison, WI
53707-7895, or visit the IVCF website at www.intervarsity.org.*

Scripture quotations, unless otherwise noted, are from the New Revised Standard Version of the
Bible, *copyright 1989 by the Division of Christian Education of the National Council of the
Churches of Christ in the USA. Used by permission. All rights reserved.*

*While any stories in this book are true, some names and identifying information in this book may
have been changed to protect the privacy of individuals.*

Cover design: Cindy Kiple
Interior design: Beth McGill
Images: ©Ebru Sidar/Trevillion Images

ISBN 978-0-8308-3594-2 (print)
ISBN 978-0-8308-9707-0 (digital)

Printed in the United States of America ∞

Library of Congress Cataloging-in-Publication Data
A catalog record for this book is available from the Library of Congress.

P 19 18 17 16 15 14 13 12 11 10 9 8 7 6 5 4 3 2 1

Y 29 28 27 26 25 24 23 22 21 20 19 18 17 16 15 14

Dedicated to all whose world has been shaken—

especially those suffering with Parkinson's

or other debilitating diseases

Contents

I am Glandion.
I am a contemplative.
I embrace the life and role of the Holy Spirit.
I love a good wine.
I love fellowship and friendships.
I am a deep, caring person.
I am a worrier and a burden bearer.
I take time to notice.
I am soft-spoken yet strong in spirit.
I love jazz, as well as the Gregorian chant.
I am consciously aware of my sinful nature.
I am a great listener.
I am a priest, a husband and father of four adult children.
I am a grandpa, affectionately called "Papa."
I long to remain in the presence of God.
I like to celebrate.
I don't have to act in a cultural manner to define my African
    American identity.
I am a crosscultural man.
I think about my death about once a week.
I think about my life and want to do the things that matter.
I love to laugh yet I cry easily.
I love poetry, especially T. S. Eliot and Garrison Keillor.
I love coffee.
I question myself all the time.

I have never sensed the condemnation of God.
I don't think about former accomplishments as much as my failures.
I believe in justice.
I have stood in lines in Ethiopia with the hungry and the poor.
I have traveled to eastern Africa during the time of genocide,
    war and famine.
I minister in one of the wealthiest communities in the United States.
I have learned that the rich in resources can also be poor in spirit.
I embrace the Scriptures and see them as a guidepost for life.
I have struggled to accept the diagnosis of a disease and tried to
    cover it up.
I love the Father, Son and Holy Spirit.
I love the Eucharist.
I embrace another person's heart, whatever their religious practice.
I believe evil will be overcome.
I love to see the sunset.
I take time to look in the eyes of others to get a glimpse of their heart.
I like to raid the cookie jar in the middle of the night.
I love theological discussions.
I am loved.
I am loving.
I am Glandion.
I have Parkinson's.
I am learning to walk in grace.

FOREWORD

⁂

IT FEELS LIKE A STRANGE COINCIDENCE—perhaps even providence—that I am writing these words at Calvin College in Grand Rapids, Michigan. It was here many years ago that I first met Glandion Carney. Back then Glandion was a church planter for the Christian Reformed denomination. He had just started up an innovative ministry, Centerpointe, which sought to bring spiritual formation into Christlikeness into every aspect of congregational life. The entire effort was bristling with vitality and life.

We were instantly drawn toward each other even though our backgrounds were vastly different. Glandion grew up in the San Francisco Bay Area in the heyday of the black power movement, and I have always appreciated the cutting-edge social concern those early years instilled in him. Of course, the Afro had long since disappeared; indeed, Glandion was quite bald when we first met. No matter. We connected deeply.

We traveled together to various places, Glandion and I, ministering the life-giving news of Jesus alive and present among his people. Together we went to England as a ministry team. British folk were instantly taken by this soft-spoken African American who embodied a special combination of dignity, grace and strength. In the northeast of England we visited Cuthbert's Cave, where the saint's body was carried by the monks from Holy Island fleeing from the Viking invaders. We hiked together in the Kyloe Hills with the north wind tugging hard at our coats and the North Sea crashing on the rocks below. On one rainy hike Glandion got a shoe stuck so deeply in the mud that his foot came out and he had to sit in the mud digging out his lost shoe. I laughed at the comical scene until my sides ached.

In those days Glandion was a model of strength and courage. He remains strong and courageous today, but in a very different way. You see, Glandion has Parkinson's disease. Nowadays he struggles even to button his shirt or to stand without falling. In unsparing detail he shares the story with us in *The Way of Grace*. At one point he writes, "No matter how old you are or how many degrees you have or don't have—when grace takes you to school, you start in kindergarten."

This is a book about grace, God's "amazing grace." To be sure, the context within which Glandion shares his experience of grace is Parkinson's disease, which is debilitating in virtually every detail of his life. But it is not a sad or disheartening book. On the contrary, while taking us deeply into the wounds of Parkinson's,

The Way of Grace is also richly refreshing. It is, as Glandion puts it, a "chosen path" in the midst of life's circumstances.

Grace is God's favor, God's gift, God's wonder-filled care for us. In this particular context it is God working with Glandion to enable him to do what he simply could not do on his own.

In rare times grace falls upon us by divine fiat. When this happens doxology is our only appropriate response. However, the most common way God imparts his grace to us is through an interactive, cooperative relationship in which God and we are working together. The reason this is grace is that the results are always in excess of the effort we put in. God works with us and alongside us, enabling us to do what we could never do in our own strength.

One reason this is God's customary means of imparting his grace to us is that through this process something quite amazing happens, something quite beyond the specific need or task at hand. Slowly, over time and experience, we become the friend of God. Step by step, we grow accustomed to God's presence. We begin entering a with-God kind of life.

Now, this "with-God kind of life" immerses us into a hidden reservoir of divine love and power, bringing into our lives God's divine life, God's *zōē*. This *zōē* life from God is unquenchable and indestructible. It is, in truth, "eternal life" as the Bible says. It has a principle of its own. No one owns it but God alone. And God graciously imparts his divine *zōē* life to us more and more as we become immersed into this "with-God kind of life." In time, this *zōē* life from God forms us into communities of grace that are enabled to express God's life and love through our own lives, individually and corporately.

In *The Way of Grace* we discover the multiplied ways this *zōē* life from God enters Glandion Carney's daily experience and sustains him. Indeed, it causes him to become "more than [a conqueror] through him who loved us" (Romans 8:37) and encourages us to do the same. It is a story of great grace in the midst of great need. "*Tolle lege*, take and read."

Richard J. Foster

1

FACING REALITY

The Grace of Acceptance

IT HAPPENED SO FAST—my body wouldn't cooperate with my mind. Never had I struggled with such simple things. I seemed to be all thumbs as I put on my clerical collar. It wouldn't go on straight no matter what I did. My jacket got stuck halfway on; it felt like a straightjacket, binding my arms and preventing me from moving correctly. What was going on? Why was I suddenly so clumsy?

It was 2008, and I was leading a pastors' conference in Kigali, Rwanda, walking men from many countries through steps of meditation, reflection and communion with God. During my trip to Africa, I had become increasingly tired, more so than I had ever been in the past. The work was grueling and the hours were long, but I had done this before and it had never bothered me. It felt like my thoughts were being stolen from my mind. I would begin a sentence and then midway I would not know where the thought was going.

My good friend William Wilson had gone along to minister with me. A former Trappist monk, he was now an Anglican priest like me. William noticed how sluggish and stiff my movements were becoming. At his encouragement I decided to go to the doctor for a physical when we got home. It seemed logical that I had picked up a virus or other illness while traveling.

My physician did his usual examination, but then asked me to do simple movements like walk a few steps and bend at the waist. He inspected my arms, knees and legs, and tested my reflexes. He shined a light in my eyes and then said simply, "You have Parkinson's disease."

Stunned, I questioned him. "How do you know? How can you say 'You have Parkinson's' when you've done no test or bloodwork to determine this diagnosis?"

He looked me straight in the eyes and responded, "You are not smiling like you used to, and your face looks frozen in a frown. Your movements are difficult. Your joints are in pain. All this points to Parkinson's. You can get a second opinion from a neurologist, but he will tell you the same thing."

Words escaped me. I felt nothing. I was empty. Numb.

There was no brilliant logic to apply. There were no prayers to pray. There was no believing or trusting in God for the future of my life in general or my ministry. All was blank, as if erased. I walked out of his office in a fog. When I got to my car I wept like a baby, leaning on the steering wheel for support. I called my wife and told her. "The doctor says I have Parkinson's."

Marion dropped what she was doing at work and came home to sit with me in silence. That's when feeling nothing moved to darkness and hopelessness. Like Job and his friend in Scripture, we sat in the ash heap of despair.

At that point I couldn't see any applications of grace. No Bible verses immediately came to mind to soothe my dark and foreboding spirit. The words "you have Parkinson's disease" played over and over in my mind like a record stuck on a track. I felt sabotaged. Tears of hurt, grief and fear fell unceasingly. I couldn't stop them if I tried.

Many saints through the centuries have referred to tears as a gift:

> The "gift of tears" written about by the desert elders and several centuries later by St. Ignatius of Loyola are not about finding meaning in our pain and suffering. They do not give answers but instead call us to a deep attentiveness to the longings of our heart. They continue to flow until we drop our masks and self-deception and return to the source of our lives and longing. They are a sign that we have crossed a threshold into a profound sense of humility.[1]

I couldn't come up with any longing in my heart, except for this new diagnosis to be recalled. It was easier to deceive myself with the drug of denial than to begin the hard work of acceptance.

A DIFFERENT DIRECTION

The physician recommended I seek physical therapy. He reminded me this disease would take its toll over time; to slow the process I needed to change my lifestyle. Get more rest. Exercise more. Start medication. Eat well. It was all so overwhelming.

When I got up the courage, I made an appointment with the physical therapist. I walked into the rehab hospital not knowing what to expect. I was blown away. Hunchbacked patients, shaking violently, were straining to remain balanced while they walked. Most were suffering with the visible effects of Lou Gehrig's disease, multiple sclerosis or Parkinson's. So many diseases and disabilities were represented—you name it and they had it. I saw myself in them and I was scared.

When the therapist called my name, I jerked to attention. Instead of following him into the therapy session, I ran out of the waiting room in tears. I left and did not go back for a year. I have never confessed this to anyone before now.

This was not supposed to be my journey. How could I face it?

I had no direction or sense of destination. I didn't even have a compass. The nothingness I had felt earlier turned into a dark shadow of gray with shades of anger. I was on a journey with no end in sight, not one I wanted, anyway. Severe difficulties had suddenly been thrust on me, and they hovered over my head like darkening clouds in a storm. Questions tormented me: Will I die? Where is God in the midst of this? Where is my courage?

I went to see a neurologist who was also a member of our

church. After he confirmed the diagnosis, he explained that Parkinson's is a disorder of the brain that leads to shaking and difficulty with walking, movement and coordination, and it continues to get worse. Seeing the immediate tears in my eyes, he came to my side, took me by the hand and said, "Just pray, Glandion. God will show you the way."

Even after two doctors confirmed the diagnosis, it took me twelve months to accept it. During that year, I concealed my difficulties. Even though my wife studied to learn more about the disease, I refused to do so. I hid out like a fugitive. I denied everything. I foolishly thought that if I didn't acknowledge the symptoms they would just go away.

One Sunday morning I was shaving in preparation for church when I heard these words in my heart: "Glandion, you don't trust me. You say you do, but you don't. You masquerade and cover up your weaknesses. You hide because you will not accept what I have allowed."

It was Jesus speaking to my heart at the deepest level. It wasn't a harsh rebuke; it was a gentle voice asking me to admit my weakness and come to the truth.

That morning I stood before my congregation as associate pastor and spoke these words: "As your priest, today I need to make a confession. I have Parkinson's disease. I have been covering up my weakness, and I need to share it openly. I'm trying to accept it as a grace. I hope you will pray for me."

Many came up afterward to speak to me: "My weakness is

drug addiction," "My weakness is pornography," "My weakness is controlling others," "My weakness is alcoholism." We wept together, held by a powerful cord of acceptance and confession.

The spiritual director in me wanted to sit down with each of them over a cup of coffee to validate their experiences of integrity, honesty and true confession. You see, my conviction is that we don't walk alone on the path of faith. We explore it together, learning about grace, trials and new beginnings. We may have different paths on the journey, but we all end at the same destination—the discovery of God's faithfulness in whatever we face.

But how could I express this truth to them when I had not experienced it myself? I admitted my weakness and began to accept it. Now I had to act on it. It was the first step to healing and freedom. There would be many others.

A year after I initially visited that rehab hospital, I returned for physical therapy. This time I knew what to expect, and I was ready to do the work. Now what I noticed in the other tormented bodies was not their dysfunction but their *eyes*. Their eyes conveyed hope, courage and a will to overcome. The grace of acceptance allowed me to see them in a different light. Instead of running away from these fellow sufferers, I was motivated to join them. And I was moved to offer up deep prayer for them as a sign of accepting our common experience.

Another turning point in this journey of acceptance was the night my wife and I ate dinner at the home of my coauthor, Marjean Brooks, and her husband, Ricky. After dinner they shared a video with us, saying it reminded them of Marion and me. In the video, a man was sleeping on the couch. His wife talked excitedly about a new home improvement tool as she walked up to the camera, drawing us in. She guaranteed results and encouraged all viewers to watch her demonstrate. Marion was getting interested. She needed some things done around the house and had been trying to motivate me to do them.

As the woman on the video spoke, she rolled up a catalog in her hands. When she finished her spiel, she walked over to her reclining husband, whacked his backside with the catalog and yelled, "Get yo' butt up!"

Marion and I laughed hard at that unexpected ending. In fact, that line has been a standing joke with us ever since. Afterward I felt as if I had been prompted: "Okay, Glandion, when are *you* going to 'get yo' butt up' and work on your life?"

Like the main character Much Afraid in the classic allegory *Hinds' Feet on High Places* by Hannah Hurnard, I glimpsed the journey with all its peaks, valleys and shadows. Just as Much Afraid took the hands of her companions Sorrow and Suffering, I took the first step of acceptance. Without realizing it, I had been blocking grace by refusing to be humbled. Now I made the choice to embrace a different way to live and a fresh power to love through God's empowering grace. I had no idea what lay ahead. But I was ready.

BEGINNING THE JOURNEY

In the course of Much Afraid's journey to the High Places, she faced tremendous difficulties. After each mountain was scaled or each terror was over, she would put a small stone in the pouch around her waist. They became trophies of grace, remembrances of all that the Shepherd had brought her through. In the end they were turned into beautiful jewels, placed in a crown for her to wear.

I haven't picked up stones along my journey. Instead God has shown me many different aspects of grace that have spurred me on my way. I have carried them until I am used to their weight in my backpack. They once seemed heavy, but now they are weightless. They are so much a part of me that I could not live without them. God's grace has been manifested to me in beautiful yet challenging ways. He gives this kind of grace to all of us—if we learn to recognize, accept and embrace it to live victoriously in this world.

Teresa of Ávila, a sixteenth-century Spanish mystic philosopher and Catholic saint, described the journey through different graces in her book *The Interior Castle*:

Let us imagine . . . that there are many rooms in this castle, of which some are above, some below, others at the side; in the centre, in the very midst of them all is the principal chamber in which God and the soul hold their most secret intercourse. Think over this comparison very carefully;

God grant it may enlighten you about the different kinds of graces He is pleased to bestow upon the soul. No one can know all about them, much less a person so ignorant as I am. The knowledge that such things are possible will console you greatly should our Lord ever grant you any of these favours.[2]

As I began to look differently at my circumstances, I wanted God to show me all the rooms in my castle. I especially wanted to see the principal chamber where he and I could hold the most secret intercourse. And I was anxious to be enlightened about the grace he would bestow.

JESUS, FULL OF GRACE AND TRUTH

On this journey into grace, I was led to see Jesus as one who both gave and modeled grace in his earthly life. It started with his acceptance to come to this world. Philippians 2:6-8 speaks of his willingness to be humbled and to empty himself of the rights of heaven in order to take his assignment on earth. Chris Tiegreen has explained this truth by writing, "Jesus went from heavenly riches to earthly rags, from exaltation to humiliation, from authority to obedience, from ultimate significance to ultimate rejection, from comfort to hardship, from safety to danger, from glory to sacrifice, and from life to death. And he calls us to go into the world *in exactly the same way!*"[3]

Jesus' acceptance and obedience brought about the saving

grace of God. Grace is simply God's unmerited favor. In other words, he gives us what we don't deserve (grace) and doesn't give us what we do deserve (judgment) because of Jesus' death on the cross. But it's more intimate than that: Grace is God's blessing overflowing into our lives. To experience God's grace is to open gift upon gift of comfort, companionship and empowerment. In his grace God saves us, strengthens us and sanctifies us. He freely offers us the gift of grace, but we must accept it.

We celebrate grace and thank God for the liberating power that comes to us through it. But it doesn't stop there—there are other aspects of grace God longs to show us. The foreword to the participant's guide of Max Lucado's book *Grace* reads: "We know *grace* as a noun, but Max tells us to think of *grace* as a verb. It is an action. It's not enough to read about grace; we must experience it."[4]

When he came to earth, Jesus was "full of grace and truth" (John 1:14). And if we, as believers, have accepted him into our lives, then "from his fullness we have all received, grace upon grace" (John 1:16). If Jesus is full of grace and truth, and he is in us, then we too can experience lives full of grace and truth. What a privilege!

The "way of grace" is the phrase I have used to describe the journey. Whether we embark on this road is up to us. It can be the chosen path or a rejected course. God offers it freely and openly. He will not force it on us.

God issues an invitation to venture to a new land. It is much like the children of Israel journeying to the Promised Land. There are dangers and giants in this foreign country, but there are also mysteries to be revealed and provisions along the way that only God can give. The invitation is to cross over into the land of grace. The question is: Will we go?

THE GRACE OF ACCEPTANCE

This book is simply a recounting of the grace God has worked in my life. Each chapter will highlight a different dimension of grace, much like the facets of a diamond. My prayer is that as you read you will find a new way to see the grace that is being offered in your own life, whatever your place of difficulty may be.

We start with the grace of acceptance (chapter one), for it was the first step of many in letting go of the control I thought I had. For me, it became a three-step process of acceptance, submission and relinquishment (continued in chapters two and three). The grace of acceptance is not a new concept but one that must be experienced before moving on. God's coming alongside to extend grace, not just once but every day, humbles me as he pours out grace upon grace. Acceptance is simply this: I receive God's invitation or offer and willingly embrace what he gives. I come to terms with the fact that I don't have all the answers. I accept his gift of grace even when it comes alongside illness, weakness or death. I move from a place of depression, self-pity and denial into the grace of acceptance.

This is what I might have become had I not experienced this grace:

- an alcoholic, abusing a substance in order to find peace
- a bad husband, seeking mental and emotional health from others while neglecting my wife
- a disbelieving priest, all the while acting out the role of a life lived in faith

Acceptance changed everything.

- Instead of thinking about death, I began to embrace life.
- Instead of ignoring people who were handicapped, I prayed for them.
- When I needed help, I asked for it, even from strangers.
- Instead of hiding, I tried to live openly and honestly about my condition.
- Even though I still had tears, I welcomed laughter.
- Instead of being afraid to open up to others, I relished deep, honest relationships.

It was revolutionary.

Grace enlarges the capacity of our heart. It allows us to be guided into truth. It gives us courage to accept and a reason to celebrate, and opens our eyes to glimpse wonders from God. The foundation for experiencing this unique call is the knowledge that we are saved by grace, live by grace and are filled with grace if we are in relationship with God through Jesus.

I talked with Christian philosopher and friend Dallas Willard about my struggle to understand grace. He leaned his tall frame toward me, gazed at me with his deep blue eyes and said, "Grace, you know, doesn't have to do with forgiveness of sins alone. Grace is for *all of life.*"

Another friend, Richard Foster, told me: "What happens after grace? Is there anything after grace? The answer is no; there is just grace." The greatest thing I want to experience and pass on to others is the reality and totality of God's grace: How to apply it to any situation and be nurtured and empowered by it. It is greater than we could ever imagine.

REFLECTION

What about you? What is the circumstance or difficulty that is hard for you to embrace? It may look completely different from mine, but no one gets through life without a cross to bear, a thorn to embrace or a difficulty to overcome.

I heard a unique story while traveling in Africa with a Bedouin tribe. It goes back hundreds of years. Two Bedouin men were traveling in the desert and came across a man who had died at an oasis. One man asked, "How could he have died—he's right at the oasis? There is shade to cover his body and plenty of water to drink." The other man replied, "He died out of fear. What he thought was a mirage was, in fact, reality."

Let us not miss the waters of grace, or faint beside them. They are not a mirage but true waters of refreshment and life. As the prophet Jeremiah wrote:

> Blessed are those who trust in the LORD,
>> whose trust is the LORD.
> They shall be like a tree planted by water,
>> sending out its roots by a stream.
> It shall not fear when the heat comes,
>> and its leaves shall stay green;
> in the year of drought it is not anxious,
>> and it does not cease to bear fruit. (Jeremiah 17:7-8)

APPLICATION

Take five minutes to sit quietly and reflect. To begin, meditate on John 1:14, 16. "And the Word became flesh and lived among us, and we have seen his glory, the glory as of a father's only son, full of grace and truth." "From his fullness we have all received, grace upon grace."

Meditate on the phrases "Jesus, full of grace and truth" and "grace upon grace." Say them over and over in your mind. Think of them throughout the day when life becomes demanding. Let the words become waters of refreshment overflowing into your life.

Pray a simple prayer:

Jesus, I thank you for your grace. May you impart your gifts to me. Help me to recognize them and to apply your grace in every situation. Grant me the grace of acceptance for what I'm struggling with today. Amen.

2

Experiencing the Presence

The Grace of Submission

As I walked down the hallway to my office, I thought about the Eucharist I would serve in a few hours. It bothered a place in my spirit like the throbbing a splinter causes in your finger.

God impressed upon me that the sacramental duty required examination, mental and physical preparation, and meditation on the act itself. Instead of preparing, I was concentrating on what it would take for me to perform the duties. It required great stamina just to go through the entire process of reading, praying and offering the elements of communion. With these concerns in the forefront, I worried. Would I lean to the right or to the left? Would I drop the communion wafers? Would I have an attack and lose the ability to keep air in my diaphragm? Would I have enough strength to finish the Eucharist?

I was extremely stiff that Sunday morning. The Parkinson's was making my body sore and causing me to shuffle and stumble. I felt as if I would fall at any moment. And being tired didn't help. I had missed the pattern of a normal week due to travel and had come home spent. I was like a boxer in the ninth round, ready to say to my opponent, "You win."

These thoughts were chasing themselves around and around in my mind as I stepped up to the altar. I stumbled, and my heart pounded. I obsessed, wondering, *Who's watching? Did anyone catch my stumble? What will they think? My church family knows about my disability, but what about visitors? Will I embarrass my community of faith?* The more I concentrated on my inadequacies, my shortcomings and my illness, the more I felt removed from the spirit of the sacrament itself.

I spoke to the congregation: "I have Parkinson's. Therefore if I lean too much to the right or the left, it's not because I've had too much communion wine."

They laughed. I felt at home.

A newly ordained deacon named Andrew stood by my side and prayed over me. He placed a stool up front for me to sit on, and he held the communion plate for me. Sometimes my fingers cramped, preventing me from being able to separate the wafers, so he also did this for me. He stood by my side the entire time as I handed the elements to each person who came to the altar, and while I pronounced words of blessing and affirmation over them.

At the altar, the Lord showed me a truth. The more I concentrated on my disease, the more removed I was from joining in the mystical experience of breaking the bread and serving the wine. But the more I submitted to Jesus *in* this broken body—in the stumbling and stiffness, in reading the liturgy with stammering lips—the more his presence became magnified. My identification with Christ became crucial; his broken body was ministering through my broken body. When I went back to concentrating on my shaky performance because of the disease, his presence subsided.

I began to see that Jesus was real and that he was next to me, even in my limited physical ability. I felt something holy, pure and righteous enter into my spirit—*a fellowship of suffering and compassion.* I didn't manufacture this or dream it up. A mysterious thing happened during the Eucharist; my physical limitations became less important and, in a simple way, I saw the love of God for every person who came forward.

Everyone who came to communion that day seemed to receive a personal word of encouragement straight from the heart of Jesus though my words. I saw glimpses into every heart as they approached the altar. Some were sincere, honest people who needed to know that Jesus loved them in a special way. Others wanted encouragement or an affirmation of God's love for them. I could see their authentic hunger for God. I looked in their eyes and saw tears as burdens were lifted.

Instead of speaking the usual words, "the body of Christ,

given for you," I said to a young man, "You have been a compassionate father to your children. God is going to be a compassionate father to you." There were tears in the eyes of an older man with a hard, sun-scorched face. For years he had been unable to connect with God and others. "God loves you more than you can ever realize," I encouraged him. To another I said, "God delights in you, you make him smile." A woman who had been healed of cancer and had returned to work heard, "Child, delight yourself in God. He is the source for all your life."

I can only explain this as a supernatural experience, which was not uncommon to the early church fathers as they administered the Eucharist. Those who came to the communion table that morning said they noticed the difference. One deacon said she saw light. Others felt the presence of Christ. I realized that my physical limitations were less important than I had made them. In fact, they were inconsequential. Jesus did his healing work in the hearts of our community, in spite of me.

As I shared lunch with friends that Sunday, I asked whether the service seemed real and honest. I was still struggling with whether those things had really happened or whether I'd made a fool of myself. Their answers left me with a deep assurance that it hadn't been a hoax or self-manufactured but an act of humility and compassion. Christ had come among us, and he had chosen to use the faltering speech and stumbling steps of one of his servants. All it took was yielding to him and taking my eyes off my own limitations. This experience enacted the truth of

John the Baptist's statement, "He must increase, but I must decrease" (John 3:30), the very definition of Christian submission.

THE GRACE OF SUBMISSION

The principle of submission is woven throughout the Scriptures. Abraham obeyed God by leaving the familiar as he traveled to an unknown land, believing the amazing promise that he would have a son in his old age, and later taking that son to be sacrificed at the direction of the Lord. Moses followed some pretty crazy instructions from God, such as boldly declaring plagues on Pharaoh and leading the Israelites out of bondage into the unknown. Joseph submitted to a plan that seemed disastrous as he was sold into slavery, then rescued out of it only to be thrust into prison without cause. When the widow had nothing but one jar of oil to pay her debts, she obeyed Elisha's instructions and received more oil than she had containers to hold. David submitted to the righteous judgment of God after he sinned with a married woman. Mary allowed God to radically change her life as she supernaturally conceived and bore his son.

Of course, the ultimate example is our Lord Jesus as he submitted himself to the Father and modeled the way of submission for us. Throughout the Gospels we hear him say repeatedly, "My time has not yet come." He knew his mission and waited on the Father for the fulfillment. He yielded to the Scriptures, saying, "It is written . . ." to the questioners, the disciples, and also to the Pharisees in their deceitfulness. He summed up his life, "My food is to do the will of him who sent me and to complete his work" (John 4:34). He submitted completely.

The grace of submission has also been taught through the ages by the desert elders, third-century Christians who lived in the desert regions of Egypt. They retreated from a life of pleasure and power to be with God and to hear from him. They lived in isolation in order to concentrate on prayer, rebuking the evil presence that came against them in their devotional life. Many people heard of their deep prayer life and chose to journey into the desert to learn their way of submission.

It is difficult for us to retreat to desert spots today to seek God. Just the thought evokes images of tarantulas, dry and sunburned skin, and parched throats. But we mustn't miss the spiritual principle that was at work, calling these saints into a life of isolation and prayer. We may not receive the same calling, but the principle of spending time alone with God so that we learn to submit is applicable to us as well. We need to learn this grace of submission.

The grace given to me by God that day during the Eucharist was the grace of submission. As I yielded my body and thoughts to God, he used me to encourage others and to bless them in their faith. At that moment of yielding, I was practicing what the desert elders taught—releasing myself to God—even in a body that was uncooperative. This grace came for my own spiritual benefit in order to teach me a greater level of submission, but it also ministered to the body of Christ. It was both an individual and a corporate blessing. It demonstrated the truth in the life of Paul as God showed him, "'My grace is sufficient for you, for power is made perfect in weakness.' So, I will boast all the more gladly of my weaknesses, so that the power of Christ may dwell in me" (2 Corinthians 12:9).

So what does this grace of submission mean in our daily lives? I believe that God gives us just enough grace to help us through everything that comes our way. I also believe that grace will accomplish the specific purpose it was called to do. Once we are trained to see and recognize grace, it often surprises us. Submission ties our hearts into the heart of the Father. As we lay down our own agendas, our own perspectives and our own thoughts, we make room to receive God's agenda, perspective and thoughts. This takes time. It takes courage to submit. The grace you receive from the Trinity—Father, Son and Holy Spirit—is one that allows you to say, "Yes, I will release my own will and control in what I consider most dear and most challenging to me in exchange for your will and power in my life."

Although we may not be called on to give our lives, we experience "little deaths," as Richard Foster calls them. It is through this very submission that we engage in a blessed experience. In my story of the Eucharist, I was learning to trust God on a deeper, more intimate level. And in exchange for this submission, he gave me a great sense of peace and an ability to minister in a new dimension. I also learned that grace could accompany every area of my life, as it can with yours.

REFLECTION

Sometimes in learning to submit to God, we become aware that we really don't trust him. One way to grow in trust is to use a reflection called the Examen. St. Ignatius, a Jesuit priest in the sixteenth century, taught this technique of prayerful reflection in his *Spiritual Exercises*.[1] The Examen is an ancient practice that helps us see God's hand at work in our experience. It consists of a five-step meditation that teaches us to detect God's presence and discern his direction for us. The steps are:

1. Become aware of God's presence.

2. Review the day with gratitude.

3. Pay attention to your emotions.

4. Choose one struggle of the day and pray about it. (This might be the area of your life that needs submission.)

5. Look toward tomorrow.

One young lawyer who met with me for a year learned the value of submission through this process of prayer, contemplation and direction. He recognized that submission could be grace, empowering him to make the right choices related to family, virtues and ethics in all areas of his life and work. He eventually admitted and released to God the sore spots in his life that had been covered up since he was a teenager. The grace of submission led him into the Scriptures, a deeper prayer life and a ruthless examination of his heart. Ultimately this process led him to freedom from alcohol and a healed relationship with his father, one of the major sources of pain that drove him into addiction.

One cannot overemphasize the value of submission.

APPLICATION

Identify what grace is supporting you now in life's struggles. Put a name to it. Some examples could be the grace of courage, the grace of emotional stability, the grace of an open heart filled with kindness and truth, the grace of material provision, the grace of friendship or whatever comes to mind, from the smallest to the largest. If all you can come up with are hard things, thank God for the grace of honesty. Place your heart and mind before God and ask him to show you the grace that sustains you, replacing any negative emotions or thoughts with the identified grace. For example, if you discover bitterness in your heart, ask God to replace it with the grace of forgiveness.

Even at this moment, as I participate in writing this section of the book, I struggle. My diaphragm is weak, and I can't get enough air in my lungs. My body is stiff and uncooperative. I am tired from a lack of sleep over several nights in a row. But I am submitting my will, emotions and heart over to God. May God grant you—and me—this grace of submission in order to bring freedom and blessing.

As you examine the grace that sustains you, turn this time into a prayer of submission, inviting God into your presence and specific needs. Here is a sample prayer. It can be repeated several times throughout the day much like a meditation.

Father, Son and Holy Spirit—help me to submit. I'm afraid; help me to overcome this fear. I choose to submit in order to learn to trust you more. Amen.

3

GIVING UP

The Grace of Relinquishment

MY WORST FEAR HAD COME TO PASS. "Glandion," I
heard him say, and somehow I knew what was coming next. "I
don't think you can finish your responsibilities as a leader."

John was the conference director, but he was also my friend.
Even that bond couldn't soften the blow: "I can't depend on you
when I really need to because of your illness." Immediately I
became angry.

"John! You know what this means to me. You see what I bring
to the ministry. How can you ask me to lay it down? I think
you're letting me go under the guise that you are concerned
about my health."

He continued, "You occasionally sleep during presentations. I've had some people say that you dozed off or looked
glassy-eyed during one-on-one sessions. Glandion, I'm so

sorry to be saying this, but I'm not sure you are physically able to do this anymore."

I knew. Deep down inside I was aware that I was falling short. But I was not willing to let go of this role that gave me significance. It was extremely fulfilling and exciting. As one of the leaders who met with the pastors who were attending the annual conference, I offered spiritual direction and counsel. My life and gifts were being affirmed and acknowledged in this work, and the Lord was using me in the lives of others. The position satisfied my desire to be engaged in the lives of people from around the country and allowed me to spend time with spiritually minded friends as we reconnected each year. It also brought in extra income. All of this was threatened when the director asked me to consider leaving due to my health.

Even though I had made it known in my church, at this point I was hiding the Parkinson's from everyone else. Or I thought I was.

I tried not to let the disease's symptoms keep me from speaking, participating or offering my gifts. But you can't hide Parkinson's. It's going to tell on you. Someone is bound to notice the physical signs: trouble with speech, extreme tiredness, shaking and stumbling.

Compounding my ongoing struggle, I had just recovered from the flu before attending another conference months earlier. The medicinal cocktail of ten pills—four in the morning, two at noon, two in the late afternoon and two at bedtime—was new to my system and made me sleepy. I did find myself nodding off when meeting with people. I asked others to assist me with my meal or help me get to my room while I was using my cane. Even though I tried to maintain the appearance of normality in order to keep up with my responsibilities, I was unintentionally taking others away from their duties and causing them to be late to meetings. Unfortunately I developed cellulitis and had to be hospitalized in the middle of the conference.

I was only able to work a few days during that conference, spending the rest of the time in the hospital. It was humiliating. Several of the other conference leaders added to my embarrassment when they visited me there. The cat was suddenly out of the bag. It was like a marquee was announcing "Glandion has Parkinson's" in colored, flashing lights. I had already begun to fear that I could no longer travel and serve at these kinds of events. So when John approached me about laying my position down, my emotions unraveled. Feelings of anger, worthlessness and depression dogged my steps.

When I started in the conference ministry years earlier, I was high energy, creative, able to lead groups, teach and counsel attendees. I knew my performance was faltering now, but nothing in me wanted to lay this position down. The suggestion that I no longer be involved in this ministry was like being asked to quit breathing.

Don't get me wrong; there was good reason for the director to do this. To be honest, the travel and the intense days of ministering to others wore me out. When I got home from a conference, it took me two weeks to recover. But I was so angry and upset when John first brought up the topic of resigning that I could not rationally put all of that into perspective.

I left his office overwhelmed with questions. What do I do? Do I just go home and sulk? Do I cut off my relationship with my friend? Do I appeal to someone higher up? Or do I let it go?

I continued to fume at home. I thought of all the things I could say in response to John. I did appeal to a higher-up. I fought for all I was worth. With these actions, I told the Lord, "I need this job to make me feel productive and whole. I cannot let it go." I was getting physically worse as I went through the mental and emotional anguish. Since emotional pain can directly affect a disease, it made my symptoms even more pronounced.

Before this incident I thought I had fully accepted my circumstances and submitted all to God, but suddenly I realized I was still holding on to what was most important to me. I thought I had learned a lesson only to find there was more to learn. I was convicted that, obviously, there were even deeper things for me to relinquish.

A STILL, SMALL VOICE

When we allow it, grace steps into messy scenarios and torn relationships. It is a very bold presence.

One morning around three I woke up, troubled. I fixed some coffee and turned to the Scriptures. I was drawn to 1 Peter 5:10: "After you have suffered for a little while, *the God of all grace,* who has called you to his eternal glory in Christ, will himself restore, support, strengthen, and establish you" (emphasis added). I looked at the larger context of the passage by reading the entire book of 1 Peter and realized the main theme was suffering. Then I did a quick study on key words in the verse, such as *called, restored, supported* and *established*. The Lord showed me so strongly that he had allowed my circumstances, and he would redeem them. I felt the conviction of the Holy Spirit, showing me the cold, judgmental way I had treated my friend John.

The God of all grace enabled me to call John that day. I asked him to forgive me for going up the ranks and for making judgments against him. He responded graciously and accepted my apology. I hadn't thought about how hard it must have been for him to ask me to step down from my position.

Looking back at it now, I see things differently. I needed to be open and honest with everyone about the disease. Psalm 51:6 says that "[God desires] truth in the inward being," which challenged me to be free of deceit at the deepest level. I also saw that I needed to be exposed to something greater than myself to make it. I needed God's grace, kindness and expressions of love. This didn't happen spontaneously; it came with time. No matter how old you are or how many degrees you have or don't have— when grace takes you to school, you start in kindergarten.

I knew about grace doctrinally and, to some degree, experientially. But God wanted to take me deeper in the process of losing a position. I learned that God is merciful, kind and loving. I don't deserve what God offers or the favor he extends. Especially at this difficult time, he offered me grace, and I was humbled by it.

Thomas à Kempis wrote these words in *The Imitation of Christ*:

> Through humility you will show me what I am, what I have been, and from whence I came, for I am nothing, and did not know. If I am left to myself, then I am nothing, and all is frailty and imperfection; but if you vouchsafe a little to regard me, soon I am made strong and am filled with a new joy.[1]

Embracing this kind of humility wasn't easy. The word *relinquishment* didn't cross my mind. Letting go was an afterthought, but I was called to it just the same.

I had started the journey with acceptance, thinking it was the destination. But acceptance led to submission, and submission broadened into relinquishment. Relinquishment involves letting go of what we are holding protectively in our hands, whether it is relationships, health, control or a cherished possession. And with relinquishment comes detachment—the healthy attitude of "hands off" for things we used to grasp. We move on to God's greater plan for our lives and post a "no fishing" sign over familiar waters.

Jesus knew all about the discipline of detachment. He made the harrowing descent that relinquished heavenly privileges for a life of human limitations. He laid down his life in obedience. His last words were ones of utter abandon: "It is finished. . . . Father, into your hands I commend my spirit" (John 19:30; Luke

23:46). We will never be called to make the same sacrifice or experience relinquishment to the degree he did, but we follow his example in laying down the things God asks us to: demanding significance, defending our own position instead of submitting to change, or resisting a direction other than the one we think is best.

We need to welcome grace, this humble yet imposing presence, to explore our hearts. It is like water flowing downward from a mountaintop, becoming a mighty, rushing river. The force of the water takes everything in its path, carrying it forward. Miles and miles later, it changes into a quiet stream that flows gently through a well-worn path. When the water is calm, you drink from the abundance of God's love only to find that it is living water. That's when your deepest thirst is met. This is renewal. This is grace—the overflow of God's heart.

In my situation, I accepted the truth. I submitted my will. And finally, I relinquished all to God, including the position I desired most to keep. With his hand on my shoulder, Jesus offered the cup, and I drank from the waters of grace. My heart was made alive.

THE GRACE OF RELINQUISHMENT

Since that time, I have to pray often: *I relinquish what is paramount to me in order to receive from you, God. I do not demand my own way. I watch to see what you might bring out of pain and loss. I am wholly submitted to you.* Grace allowed God to penetrate the

depths of my soul, bringing to it the deep work of the Holy
Spirit. It awakened the dormant heart with power as faith
became interactive. Mere words turned into reality: God's grace
is sufficient for everything. Oswald Chambers said, "No one is
ever united with Jesus Christ until he is willing to relinquish not
sin only, but his whole way of looking at things."[2]

Gradually, new roles and opportunities opened up for me. For
several years I had been serving as priest in my church on a
volunteer basis, but now a salaried position was approved for me
as associate pastor. This provided income as well as benefits
(something I did not have before). I was in charge of pastoral
care, which allowed me to meet with individuals in the congregation for prayer and counseling. I also visited the homebound
and those in the hospital. As coordinator of prayer ministries, I
loved encouraging others in this vital discipline of faith. Even
more significantly, John offered a way for me to continue in the
conference program, offering spiritual direction through Skype
and FaceTime. This gracious offer allowed me to participate in
a ministry role without the pressures of traveling.

I have accepted the need to give up the public part of my
ministry. I have embraced the slower pace that gave me the opportunity to write this book, another blessing. I am no longer
thinking of my death once a week. *I am looking forward to life.* I
am pushing through outward symptoms and being healed in a
new way. I am being strengthened through physical therapy and
speech therapy. Medication is a grace to me; it allows my body

to accept the dopamine that is needed to keep me steady and strong. Only grace turned me toward this journey. I know I am receiving God's favors.

Other believers through the ages have come to the place of relinquishment. Jim Elliot, missionary to the Auca people in Ecuador, relinquished his life for the sake of the gospel. His journal entry for October 28, 1949, expresses his belief that missions work was more important than his life, famously saying, "He is no fool who gives what he cannot keep to gain that which he cannot lose."[3] God graced him with heart, passion and zeal that ultimately led to his death at age twenty-nine by the hands of the natives he came to serve. However, what seemed to be tragedy was turned to triumph as his wife, Elisabeth, returned to finish his work and to bring the gospel to the Aucas.

George Müller was a pastor from Bristol, England, in the 1800s. He was known for his deep prayer life. But hidden in this man of great faith is a life of relinquishment, as he chose to depend on God for his own needs, as well as the needs of thousands of orphans in his care. He chose to speak their needs to God alone, relinquishing completely in the hands of a gracious God. As a result, he raised more than seven billion dollars in the span of sixty years of ministry to tend to "the least of these" (see Matthew 25:31-46).

Modern-day disciples face the same difficulties. When Dallas Willard was very ill with pancreatic cancer, I called him and offered to pray with him. He had just resigned after forty years as a professor at the University of Southern California. He shared with me his own experiences of letting go in order to receive God's greater gift of grace in this season.

Even in these examples, relinquishment is not a simple struggle with an easy outcome. Jim Elliot lost his earthly life and never got to see his daughter grow up. George Müller spent a great part of his life on his knees, petitioning and arguing with God. Dallas Willard was not miraculously healed. I am still dealing with the effects of Parkinson's. But this does not stop the grace of God from invading the heart and strengthening us to do his will.

REFLECTION

Simone Weil was a French philosopher and Christian mystic in the twentieth century. In her book *Gravity and Grace* she said, "Grace fills empty spaces but it can only enter where there is a void to receive it. We must continually suspend the work of the imagination in filling the void within ourselves."[4]

This teaching goes hand in hand with the picture of the cleansing waters of grace. When we empty ourselves of our own imaginations, we open ourselves to the force of grace, just like the rushing mountain waterfall. For example, when we open our hands and offer to God the things dearest to us, we are opening ourselves to the cleansing power of grace. Even realizing we are clinging to these things is a grace! When grace pours over our lives, it moves us toward wholeness and health. It removes the contamination of the world and purifies our hearts.

What is keeping you from experiencing relinquishment? What are you grasping in clenched hands? What is holding you back? Fill in the blank with whatever you are insisting on: "Lord, I have to have _____ in order to be whole and happy."

APPLICATION

Visualize the most important things in your life right now: Your hopes, dreams, ambitions, family, friends and future. Place them symbolically in your open hands and lift them to God, relinquishing all to him. Release your need for control, your craving for status, your fear of obscurity or anything else God reveals. Ask him to take away the evil, to purify the good and to establish his kingdom in your life.

Read this verse out loud and imagine Jesus offering you the cup from which to drink: *"Let anyone who is thirsty come to me, and let the one who believes in me drink. As the scripture has said, 'Out of the believer's heart shall flow rivers of living water'"* (John 7:37-38).

Kneel in relinquishment, realizing God's provision of grace. Respond in prayer:

Dear God, cleanse me of the imaginations I've used to fill the void in my own life. I cannot receive the cup until I let go of the things I am clinging to. I relinquish all to you. I choose to drink from your waters of grace. Amen.

May God's grace wash over your soul, cleanse your heart and strengthen you to do his will.

STUCK IN AN AIRPORT

The Grace of Compassion

IT WAS A BEAUTIFUL DAY IN CHICAGO as I got off the plane. The bright sun caused reflections in the glass enclosing the terminal, and as I glanced at one of the windows, I saw a man hunched over in a wheelchair. With his hand on his head, he looked helpless and depressed. All of a sudden I realized, *That man is me!*

It was a shocking discovery. I was no longer the fit and able man running through the airport, traveling around the world feeling significant and important. Instead, I was a man dependent on someone else to take me everywhere I needed to go, even to the bathroom.

As people passed, I imagined them thinking: "I wonder what's wrong with him?" "I feel sorry for him." Or, "Why is he getting to go ahead of me?" These thoughts probably weren't accurate, but they came unbidden as I was wheeled off the flight. I felt as if a sign were pinned to my chest: "I have Parkinson's. I'm sorry."

It was the first time I had traveled since laying down my conference ministry position. Heading to Chicago to speak to the national leaders of InterVarsity Christian Fellowship's prayer and spiritual formation ministries, I felt comfortable in this role so close to my heart and looked forward to the time. But fears dogged my preparations after my last conference experience. I was concerned about having enough strength to do the event, getting sick and having to go home, and just maneuvering through the airport.

My transport parked me in a "holding place," where I was to remain until someone came to take me to the baggage area. Once in baggage, an InterVarsity staff person would pick me up, but I would be confined to my chair until my assistance arrived. In two hours, I would stand before a group of people as a conference speaker. But as I waited for my contact to come, I felt stranded. Suddenly I wanted to go home.

I remembered that it was time to take my medicine but found the process of opening and closing the bottle difficult because my fingers wouldn't cooperate. I got the top off and took the pill, but I couldn't get the cap back on. I fumbled around trying to accomplish this for about five minutes, feeling extremely conspicuous.

A man appeared in front of me. "Hello—I see you're strug-

gling to put the medicine cap back on. May I do that for you?"
I looked up at him and said, "Thank you," and I began, out of
embarrassment, to tell him why I couldn't do it.

He said with a soft voice, "My dad died ten years ago of
Parkinson-related illness. I understand." With those kind words
and his easy closing of the cap, he touched a deep place in my
heart. I saw and felt such compassion in his words and face.

"Where do you live?" I asked.

"The south of France. I'm on my way home," he said.

I told him I was a priest, on my way to a conference. He
shared that, although he was a "lapsed Catholic" and had a hard
time believing, he still had faith. At that moment, the noises in
the airport were muted as we spoke about intimate issues. Two
strangers opened their hearts to each other, both in need of help
at different levels. I needed assistance and dignity; he needed
someone to validate his faith and encourage him to trust God
on a deeper level.

After we talked for a bit, he took it upon himself to call my
contact waiting at the luggage claim, telling them I was stuck at
the gate. Finally the transport showed up to take me to baggage
and my conference contact. Before leaving me, my new friend
spoke to me in French, saying goodbye with beautiful words. I
said my own blessing to him for his kindness.

God is a God of detail, as well as a God of compassion. Out
of thousands of people in one of the busiest airports in the world,
he sent a man who would understand my need, one who noticed

I was having difficulty putting on a medicine cap. This stranger saw more than a man in a wheelchair, and through his compassion he showed me that God saw me too. When I reflected on this chance meeting, I wondered whether he was an angel.

His compassion was enough to renew my confidence to stand up and teach before a group that week. It turned out to be one of the best speaking opportunities I ever had. I was clearheaded and focused. I even used the story of my encounter in the airport as an illustration in one of my presentations.

God also showed up at another airport at another time. On a different ministry trip to Colorado, I again sat at the gate waiting for a wheelchair to arrive. I thought that no one would notice me among the other passengers waiting to get on the plane.

A woman appeared and said, "I want to carry your suitcase." I thanked her but told her I could do it myself. She wouldn't give up. She stayed by my side and walked me down the long corridor without the need of a wheelchair. When we got through the small door in the plane, she said, "Now you take my seat in 3A, and I will take yours in 13A." She guided me into her first-class, leather, oversized seat. Instead of peanuts and a soda, I dined on roasted chicken, wine, fruit and cheese along with great coffee. Rather than being cramped in a tight seat in coach, I stretched out in comfort and slept like a baby all the way to Colorado. God provided rest through the compassion of a stranger. Again, I was cognizant of the fact that he sees me—and he cares.

The grace of compassion is powerful.

THE GOD WHO SEES

Because of the compassion shown to me by these airport angels
and others, I began to look at strangers in a different way—not
for what they could do for me, but what I could offer them. As in
the saying often attributed to Plato, "Be kind, for everyone you
meet is fighting a hard battle."

Through these experiences with strangers, Jesus became even
more present to me. As our great high priest, he is compassionate toward us and aware of our frailties. Hebrews 4:15-16
says: "For we do not have a high priest who is unable to sympa-
thize with our weaknesses, but we have one who in every respect
has been tested as we are, yet without sin. Let us therefore ap-
proach the throne of grace with boldness, so that we may receive
mercy and find grace to help in time of need."

When Jesus walked the earth and ministered among the crowds,
he had compassion on the multitudes, considering them as sheep
without a shepherd (Matthew 9:36). He looked through a different
lens and quickly picked up on the suffering people. His compassion
extended to individuals who were downtrodden, as in the story of
the woman caught in adultery. With kindness and healing, he
tended to the ill, the bereaved and the untouchable. Power and
compassion even flowed out of his garments, and a woman was
healed because of her faith from the simple act of touching them.
He wept at the tomb of Lazarus, although he knew he would raise
him from the dead. His character was displayed on the cross as he
died in the most compassionate act ever recorded. He considered

the confession of another man being crucified alongside him with the words, "Truly I tell you, today you will be with me in Paradise" (Luke 23:43). And his compassion for unrepentant sinners was expressed as he uttered, "Father, forgive them; for they do not know what they are doing" (Luke 23:34). He is a compassionate Savior!

Some of these examples are of people who sought the help of Jesus. Others did not, or could not, ask Jesus for compassion. When I was confronted with an offer of help on my way to Colorado, I tried to refuse it. Jesus gave it nonetheless, because he *is* grace, and it is in his nature to be merciful. Even when you don't ask, don't know how to ask or feel too sorry for yourself *to* ask, Jesus often intervenes anyway. Can the gift of compassion grow deeper with prayer and requests to receive it? Yes! "Ask, and it will be given you; search, and you will find; knock, and the door will be opened for you" (Matthew 7:7). But does God give compassion even if you don't ask? Again, the answer is yes. "But God proves his love for us in that while we still were sinners Christ died for us" (Romans 5:8). Grace, grace and more grace.

Compassion is the deep awareness of the suffering of another coupled with the wish to relieve it. When we come to faith in Christ and receive his provision of grace and mercy in salvation, we are beneficiaries of God's great compassion. This takes humility. It takes exposing our neediness. It is often far easier to extend compassion to others than to admit our own need for it. But in receiving compassion, we can become channels of grace to others. As we grow in our relationship to God, we become more concerned about those around us, and we learn to show compassion like Jesus did.

I feel there are seven unique qualities to this grace of compassion:

- First, knowing about it and experiencing it are two different things. Ask God to give you the grace of compassion.

- Compassion will open your heart to needs beyond your ability to meet. Don't get overwhelmed by this; it is God's job to satisfy the needs, but he might use you as a conduit.

- The grace of compassion will broaden your prayer life. It takes your eyes off yourself and onto others.

- Compassion sees the sick as well as the healer. We can be both at different times.

- Compassion reveals an intimate part of God's character. We know him as *El-roi*, "the God who sees" (a Hebrew name of God found in Genesis 16:13).

- Receiving and extending compassion will leave you humble.

- The grace of compassion has a language all its own. It is spoken with deeds of kindness, acts of mercy and being fully present in the sufferings of others.

THE GRACE OF COMPASSION

I know many who have been touched by this grace. Andy Russell, a thirty-seven-year-old trained in mechanical engineering, changed his course to become a full-time Christian worker with Compassion International. His story begins with stepping into the sewers of Romania because he heard children were living under the streets. Carrying twenty lunches, he felt compelled to enter their world. As he removed the manhole cover, he descended into a life of suffering he never knew existed. The lunches were a small token of compassion that eventually led to him working with a worldwide ministry whose focus is to release children from poverty in Jesus' name.

Andy feels that, in order to have compassion for someone else, you must put yourself in his or her place. The Latin word for compassion is *compati*, which means "to bear or to suffer." Reaching out in compassion often calls us to sacrifice our time, money or actions on behalf of others. It enables us to step outside what the world calls us to—ego-driven, materialistic, narcissistic self-gratification. It causes us to be focused on people, not on physical things. The ultimate fruit of compassion is being blessed ourselves. Jesus said, "Blessed are the merciful [or compassionate], for they will receive mercy" (Matthew 5:7).

Showing compassion is like exposing darkness to light. Once good has been introduced to an evil structure, it draws attention to the need for change. One could say, "What good will a few lunches do in combating pervasive hunger and poverty?" As this story shows, the light exposed the darkness and began a life-changing process for both Andy and hundreds of thousands of children in the world. He is just one worker among thousands in the battle against childhood poverty, but his contribution is significant and eternal.

Years ago I traveled to Ethiopia during a civil war. One morning I awoke to a strange wailing. I got dressed and walked up a hill to where thirty women were marching in a circle, carrying large stones that represented their burdens lifted to God. The lead woman clutched a dead baby who appeared to be about three months old. The infant had died from malnutrition and hunger. Leaving that scene with a heavy heart, I walked down the hill to find thousands of people standing or lying around. About three hundred waited to see a doctor who would treat their illnesses; the others were there to receive food. There was total silence except for an occasional cough or crying baby. A lone white doctor tended to all the patients; his light skin stood out in contrast to the caramel-colored Ethiopians.

I was struck by the compassion of this doctor as he patiently examined each person and decided who would go to the hospital. While he stood in the hot, baking sun, he ministered with a gentle touch and words of encouragement. Finding out he was from Seattle, I realized he could have been in the comfort of his own home or sitting on the wharf having a cup of the city's great coffee. Instead, he was ministering to the hungry, sick and war-ravished people in an African country.

He invited me to walk along the triage line as he handed out fifty slips of paper to those who would receive extended care. Only the pregnant and the sickest among them would be chosen.

My eyes welled with tears as I saw children with extended bowels and bloated stomachs. The mothers were thin and malnourished themselves, unable to feed their children.

I asked the doctor, "What can *I* do?"

He responded, "You can pray. Touch them and pray for them."

I felt so helpless. What could I say to help relieve their suffering? I prayed to the God of compassion, who cares for each of them. "God, please bless them, nourish them and sustain them." This scene forever changed me. It opened my heart, left a lasting imprint on my spirit and broadened my capacity to love.

Catherine of Siena was another example of the grace of compassion. As a baby, she was spared from the ravages of the Black Plague in the 1300s. This horrid disease killed a third of Europe in three years. Later, as a nun of the Dominican Order, she became a nurse and saved many plague victims through her compassionate care. Her bed was a board and her pillow was a log. Her only possession was a crucifix, and she identified with Christ through her attention to the sick and the poor. She believed in "mysticism in action" and worked day and night in great compassion with her patients. For Catherine of Siena, prayer was the calling into the compassionate life: "You are rewarded, not according to your work or your time, but according to the measure of your love."[1]

REFLECTION

Compassion can be awakened through prayer and by an increased love for God. It is one of the most significant aspects of grace we can receive because it so closely ties us in to the heart of the Father. If we get too involved in the tasks of our daily lives, we could miss the opportunity for compassion. We must retrain our hearts to listen, observe and pay attention to those around us who are in need of a special touch.

My cowriter, Marjean, shared a song with me that she wrote during a refining process. I believe the words can be helpful in shifting our focus off ourselves and onto others.

Tears in a Bottle

God has put all my tears in a bottle,
And he has kept them there for a long, long time—
He has put my tears in a bottle and
    Covered it with love,
He has put my tears in a bottle for you.

He captured all my heartaches in that bottle,
And not a single tear has missed his gaze—
All the prayers and the petitions
    I've offered in those days,
He has put my tears in a bottle for you.

You ask, "What's the purpose of that bottle?"
Well friend, the mystery to me has been revealed—
For when you tell me of your heartache
    And ask how I can smile,
He has put my tears in a bottle for you.

For he nurtured *the oil of gladness* in that bottle
And made the *spirit of compassion* in it, too.
And now I comfort you with that lotion—
    The way he's done for me—
He has put my tears in a bottle for you.

For he nurtured *the oil of gladness*
And *the spirit of compassion,*
And the way he's comforted me, I now comfort you.
I just reach for that bottle
    And pour out his love . . .
That's why he kept that bottle, just for you.[2]

APPLICATION

Pause for a moment and meditate on Jesus' life and his compassion for others. Recall a story from the Bible where you witnessed him showing compassion. What unique qualities in the story point to your own need for his touch?

Identify where the grace of compassion is stifled or not flowing in your own life. Turn this need into a prayer. Imagine Jesus standing near as you open your heart to him. Receive his compassion and ask for the grace to extend it to others.

Pray this prayer from Mother Teresa:

Lord, open our eyes
That we may see you in our brothers and sisters.
Lord, open our ears

That we may hear the cries of the hungry,
The cold, the frightened, the oppressed.
Lord, open our hearts
That we may love each other as you love us.
Renew in us your spirit.
Lord, free us and make us one.
Amen.[3]

God Is Not Mad at You

The Grace of Trust

✵

What happens after disaster strikes or when the storm passes with destruction in its wake? What is our response after the diagnosis is given, the time of death is confirmed or the relationship officially severed? In cases like these, the initial sense of shock is often replaced by a deep sense of grief or despair.

In the opening chapter, I wrote about receiving the diagnosis of Parkinson's, but I didn't go into my struggle the following year. Those were dark days, a time of intense discouragement, doubt and anger toward God. I am opening them up to you now as a confession.

Is This the Way You Treat Your Servant?

Before I went to the doctor with my difficulties, a good friend and former colleague tried to convince me that I had Parkinson's.

He imitated the way I walked and mocked me, saying I was an embarrassment. So when I received the diagnosis with no hope of a cure, a great sense of shame kept me from telling others.

About this same time I was ordained as a priest in the Anglican Church. (After joining St. Peter's in Birmingham I felt led to become officially connected to the denomination by becoming a priest. I had formerly been a pastor and church planter in the Reformed Church.) At my ordination people asked, "What's going on with you, Glandion?" "Are you okay?" "How's your health?" I know they were probably genuinely concerned, but I was defensive and hurt by their comments and probing questions.

Like going into a dark tunnel, I began to withdraw into isolation from God and others. Along with this coping mechanism, I was also in a very dry season in my devotional and prayer life. By "dry" I mean that God seemed far off, as if he had removed his presence from me. There is a saying, "When God seems far away, guess who's moved?" I knew it was my fault, but it didn't keep me from feeling like an orphan, abandoned and forgotten.

During this painful period I spoke at a conference in Menlo Park, California. At the same time my mother was dying thirty miles away in Oakland. In retrospect I shouldn't have been traveling and speaking; I should have been with my dying mother or at home in Alabama. When I don't trust God I keep up many fronts and pretend that all is well. My mother died a month later. Grief over her passing exacerbated my illness, making the symptoms of fatigue and stumbling even worse.

I vacillated between being mad at God and wondering whether he was mad at me. At times it felt like both were true. I might never have thought about God being angry with me if I hadn't developed this serious illness.

I was drowning in the poison of self-pity. For the next nine months this preoccupation with myself drove me away from God, my family and others who loved me. Some days my self-indulgence felt warm and comforting. Other days I was chilled by its jeering condemnation. I began thinking about my death and planning for my funeral at least once a week. Instead of living in the present and going to God with these miseries, I comforted myself with the pain, but it never brought lasting relief—only more despair. God let me have my pity party until I was tired of it. He waited patiently and then said, "Are you ready to come out now and talk?"

I also dulled my pain and soothed my sorrow by drinking too much alcohol. An evening glass of wine or one vodka and lime soon turned into two, then three or more. The alcohol loosened my tongue, releasing the pent-up anger inside: "God, is this the way you treat your servant? *If so, I don't want to be your servant!*"

My father and brother had been delivered from alcoholism. I thought I was immune because of my faith, but here I was, walking into the possibility of addiction because of physical and emotional pain. Everything I counseled others not to do, I was doing. I was a hypocrite.

As I realized this, regret flooded my heart. I wept, confessing my sin to God. Even though I knew he didn't like what I was doing, I never felt condemned. I confessed my drinking to my pastor. I met with another friend whom I had helped walk away from dependency on alcohol, telling him of my struggle. I made myself accountable to both men and asked for help. My pastor encouraged me to pray through Psalm 23 every day for a month, focusing on the first verse, "The LORD is my shepherd, I shall not want."

I also saw how alcohol abuse could lead to other sins. It unmasked my raw self, brought temptation to lust, fueled doubt and gave false courage. By depending on it as a surrogate, it stopped me from throwing myself on God for help and comfort. I have been vigilant not to overindulge ever since.

I'm embarrassed by this story because there is no hero or tough man rising up in strength and victory. I needed time to heal and process my emotions without judgment or shame. Jesus was patient with me, and I needed to be patient with myself. A theological understanding of God's anger and my own sin was not what I needed at a time of great pain. It is good to have that foundation, but when there is an emotional earthquake, everything is on shaky ground. Just as in the biblical account of Job, I found that God answers as we seek him, even if it is with more questions. The answers to the devastation in Job's life were not given; instead, an affirmation of God's sovereignty was revealed as Job sat in the ash heap of despair.

The stories in the Bible represent the gamut of human behavior, exposing our frailty: Abraham lying on two occasions, saying Sarah was his sister; Sarah laughing when the angel told Abraham they would have a child at their advanced age; Jacob and his conniving ways in stealing the birthright from his brother; Moses and his reticence to take on a mission because he was not eloquent of speech; Peter jumping out of a boat only to sink when he didn't keep his eyes on the Lord; Paul murdering and terrorizing Christians before his own conversion; Thomas doubting that Jesus had truly risen from the dead. The list goes on and on.

If these individuals had publicists, I'm sure they wouldn't have wanted them to talk about their shortcomings. Possibly they would have been encouraged to tell the truth, just not the whole truth. Thankfully the failings *and* the triumphs are recorded for our instruction. It was especially helpful for me to learn that *biblical characters are not models for morality but rather mirrors for identity.*[1] Through their stories, we see our own hearts. We can learn from their struggles and failings and know that we are not alone. This gives us courage when we realize, like the comic-strip character Pogo, "We have met the enemy, and the enemy is us."

ABANDONED BY GOD?

So how do we deal with the hand we are dealt? How do we walk through painful circumstances with the understanding that God's attributes have not changed: he is still sovereign, he is still loving, and he is still merciful and filled with grace. Is God indeed mad at us?

We see God's anger throughout the Old Testament. He was angry with Pharaoh when he refused to let his people leave Egypt. He was angry when the children of Israel made the golden calf and worshiped in the wilderness. He was angry when the Israelites were unfaithful to him. But he did not "wash his hands" of them because of their sin, refusing to hear their cries or abandoning them in the wilderness.

I believe today he is angry over the way we treat the world and one another, over poverty, child abuse, racial injustice and religious hypocrisy. But his righteous anger does not lead to him being mad, acting as a vengeful God arbitrarily inflicting suffering and placing illnesses on his people. He tempers his anger with mercy. Psalm 103:8 says:

> The LORD is merciful and gracious,
>   slow to anger and abounding in steadfast love.
> He will not always accuse,
>   nor will he keep his anger forever.
> He does not deal with us according to our sins,
>   nor repay us according to our iniquities.
> For as the heavens are high above the earth,
>   so great is his steadfast love toward those who fear him;
> as far as the east is from the west,
>   so far he removes our transgressions from us.

Throughout history, God's anger has led to righteous actions, ultimately ending in redemption and mercy.

The Bible teaches that on Good Friday God's wrath (the displeasure and indignation of the Divine against evil) was satisfied by Jesus' death on the cross. Isaiah 53:6 says, "All we like sheep have gone astray; we have all turned to our own way, and the LORD has laid on him the iniquity of us all." Jesus bore not only our sins but also God's righteous anger toward sin and rebellion, which should rightly have been placed on his fallen creatures. But the Son of God took our place and, in doing so, fully bore the wrath of God. If we are in Christ, we are no longer subject to wrath! There is nothing we need to do to appease him because, in Jesus, payment for sin has been accomplished. Therefore, things that happen in our lives are not punishment due to his anger.

Why then do sickness and suffering remain in the world today? Why do I have Parkinson's? The simple answer is that we live in a fallen world, not that God is mad at us. Our bodies are subject to illness and death. To help explain more about this difficult question, a friend of mine has allowed me to share his story.

I met Mark Ashpole years ago at a family life retreat. He was a quiet man, a pastor and a strategist from his stint in the military. I had no idea that he suffered from debilitating migraine headaches that would cause him to retreat into a dark room, sitting for hours or days until the pain subsided.

The question Mark asked during his frequent and severe

headaches was, "Where are you, God, when I'm in pain?" This is the common cry of humanity when agony is at its worst. Where is God when pain reached the level that required a trip to the emergency room? Why doesn't he answer my cries? When Mark felt abandoned by what seemed like no answer or deliverance, his eyes were opened. In his own words:

> Jesus tells us that his yoke is easy and his burden is light (Matthew 11:30). It seems straightforward to connect Christ's easy yoke with being free from pain and trouble. But Christ's way is different as we are joined to him. He doesn't always remove pain but instead shares the burden with us in going through pain. While Christ's yoke is easy, our days can still be hard and difficult.
>
> Our pain is important because it broadens our understanding of Christ's humanity and sacrifice. If Christ were exclusively divine, his suffering would seem easy to endure: A god would just call on his divine powers to ease his pain. Jesus was not only fully God but fully human and, in his humanity, he understands our pain. We are told Jesus experienced all that we do, because he was made like us in every way. He learned obedience in the midst of suffering, shared our weakness, resisted sin when tempted and was obedient even unto death (Hebrews 2:14, 17-18; 5:8; Philippians 2:8). When we feel intense pain we can know that, because of his humanity, Christ experienced worse pain on the cross.
>
> But do we really believe, deep down, in Jesus' humanity? As

a pastor, I would have said that Jesus suffered as a human suffers. But I suspect a part of me may have almost subconsciously held out that, somehow, it must have been easier for him because, well, he was Jesus and I'm just me. It took my own pain to come to grips with this subconscious falsehood. Perhaps thinking he wasn't exactly like me was a way to make me feel a little better about what my sin did to hurt Christ. It's hard to say for sure. But knowing that Jesus did hurt and suffer tells us about him and his sacrifice. When we feel pain or are afraid, lonely or abandoned, we can know that Jesus understands.

I was comforted to know that Christ understood my pain, but I was still bothered that my pain remained even when I grew in faith. I learned that Christ increased in wisdom and in stature and in favor with God and man (Luke 2:52). But this growth did not stop his [experience of] physical pain [on the cross] and, in the same way, I cannot count on God to stop all pain and hardship because I grow spiritually. I found that Christ could transform me in many ways, yet I still had headaches. In this world, spiritual renewal will not bring physical perfection, healing of all relationships or control of the presence of evil.

I found answers to my questions in this assurance: Yes, God is present and active when we are in pain. Grace allows us to live in the midst of the struggle, but it is not a metaphor for narcotics. Grace allows us to live our lives and to have hope. God's grace is that I find him in my times of pain and discover that he has not abandoned me.

This is what grace looks like in my life: a wife and two children who love me, care for me and give me reasons to live even when living with me can be hard. Grace is not just being loved but loving deeply in return. Grace is the difference between a medical staff that just prescribes medicines and those who help me plot a course to live the best possible life in spite of headaches. Grace is reading a note from someone I've never met and being told that I am loved and being prayed for.

Abandoned by God? Even though I still have pain, God has shown me that my life is too crowded to feel abandoned.

THE GRACE OF TRUST

Like Mark, the grace that ministered to me during my intense struggle was the grace of trust. First, we do have a right *not* to trust; it is a choice. But then we realize we have the opportunity *to* trust, which is a decision. God's grace is a bridge to this trust.

I had to choose to turn from the comfort that alcohol brought to trust completely in God's grace. As a result of his grace, I am stronger emotionally than when I was first diagnosed—through medication, rest, the believing prayers of others and God's continued faithfulness.

The biblical characters I discussed earlier all came to a place of trust after their shortcomings and struggles. Abraham became Father Abraham, the patriarch of the faith. Sarah had the joy of giving birth to Isaac and naming him "he laughs" in Hebrew. Jacob trusted in and wrestled with God, and as an outcome received the new name "Israel." Moses went on to become the great deliverer of his people. Peter became a stalwart leader of the early church. Thomas trusted in the truth of God's ways after seeing the Lord with his own eyes. After conversion to Christianity, Paul became the greatest apostle of all and wrote much of the New Testament. And Job uttered one of the most famous statements in the Bible: "Though He slay me, yet will I trust Him" (Job 13:15 NKJV). All were transformed because of the grace of trust.

Jesus also trusted the Father with his life, abandoning himself to the will of God. "And while being reviled, He did not revile in return; while suffering, He uttered no threats, *but kept entrusting Himself to Him who judges righteously*" (1 Peter 2:23 NASB, emphasis added). The verb used here is the imperfect tense, which means the action is ongoing and continuous. Later in 1 Peter we are encouraged as fellow sufferers to "entrust [our] souls to a faithful Creator in doing what is right" (1 Peter 4:19 NASB). If Jesus had to continually entrust himself to God, how much more do we?

The grace of trust is a firm belief in the truth of God's Word, his ability and his character. It develops over time. Just like a workout builds physical muscle, we build spiritual muscle by choosing to trust God and his goodness. For someone who has lost the ability to walk, physical therapy reprograms the body and the mind to cooperate with each other and to work in unison. As a baby step leads to several steps, and several steps gradually lead to mobility, this mobility leads to confidence in our spirits as well as our bodies. Trust in God reprograms our minds and our hearts to embrace spiritual truths, such as his love and faithfulness. It brings a daily dose of grace as we begin to see things differently. A deep-seated sense of trust leads to the acceptance of God's loving sovereignty in our life. The opposite of trust is doubt, avoiding a commitment to God by trusting in our own abilities to deliver ourselves through our own efforts.

In chapter three I spoke of drinking from the waters of grace. The grace of trust calls us to throw ourselves into these same waters. After doing this, we are immersed in the grace of God. Not only are we cleansed and refreshed, but our whole weight is buoyed and carried by his mercy and love. We find, as Deuteronomy 33:27 says, "The eternal God is a dwelling place, and underneath are the everlasting arms" (NASB).

Protestant missionary Amy Carmichael's life was an example of trusting God, even in the most severe circumstances. Originally from Ireland, she was called to serve in India in the early 1900s. Her work centered on rescuing hundreds of young girls who were "married to the gods" and used as prostitutes in the Hindu temples. She opened an orphanage to care for them and eventually opened a home for the boys who were born to these young mothers. She was both a hated figure by the religious authorities and a beloved figure to those she saved. They called her "child-catching Missy Ammai."

After a serious fall, she spent the last twenty of her fifty-five years of service confined to her room. During this time she wrote thirteen books and used her gift of writing to bring inspiration to countless readers. She worked tirelessly for the Lord, not once taking a furlough from her work. When confronted with painful or difficult things, she said, "See in it a chance to die," meaning dying to ourselves and our expectations of life.[2] Her legacy of faith includes the conviction: "It is a safe thing to trust Him to fulfill the desires which He creates."[3] To this day both the institutions she began and her writings remain. She continues to encourage others to trust a God who not only cares for children caught in physical slavery but also for those who work in obscurity due to a disability.

REFLECTION

The grace of trust requires examination. We need to ask the honest question, What am *I* trusting in? What am I depending on for day-to-day life, health and provision?

After all the discussion in this chapter and in Scripture, it is clear that the presence of pain or suffering in your life does not mean that God is mad at you. But there is another possible question: Are you mad at God? Take time to explore this idea. If you are mad, he can handle it. He already knows about it and can give you the grace to walk through your struggles with honesty.

Romans 8:28 assures us: "We know that all things work together for good for those who love God, who are called according to his purpose." This does not mean that all things *are* good but that all things will work *for* our good. Believing that, in a nutshell, is the grace of trust.

APPLICATION

We trust in a God who is characterized by this wonderful statement in Lamentations 3:22-23: "The steadfast love of the LORD never ceases, his mercies never come to an end; they are new every morning; great is your faithfulness."

Ask for the grace of trust to be strengthened in your life today. If trusting God consistently is a particular struggle, you might find a "pocket cross" and keep it near you. When you are tempted to move away from trust, hold the cross in your hand and pray a simple prayer.

Lord, I trust you with my life. Please give me the grace to trust you more in every circumstance.

May we all continue to grow in the grace of trust.

6

Wounded Healers

The Grace of Community

What does a black man from California have in common with southern whites from Alabama? When I moved to Birmingham in 1998, I would have said nothing.

I grew up in radical Berkeley, California, in the sixties. As a young person, my heroes were the Black Panthers. We shouted, "Black power!" and "Death to the system!" and despaired at the assassination of Martin Luther King Jr.

At seventeen I became a Christian through the life and witness of a high school teacher named Kenneth Jensen. A white man, he dared to venture into my ghetto neighborhood to provide tutoring for those of us who struggled in school. With his horn-rimmed glasses, wing-tipped shoes and crew cut, he was the polar opposite of the students he taught with our cool shades, black ankle boots and Afros. The most important feature about him, though, was his passionate love for God. In addition to tutoring, he helped me understand how to live a life of faith while also caring about social issues. He planted seeds of tolerance and love in me that are still bearing fruit today. He taught me to accept people for who they are, no matter their race or station in life. In other words, his legacy was one of grace.

After my conversion to Christianity in 1967, my political and social views began to evolve as I sat under dynamic preaching in an environment of Hispanics, blacks and whites worshiping together. This multicultural background helped me to embrace the banner of "equality for all" regardless of ethnicity. We understood the call for equality as well as the life-changing power of the gospel of grace found in Jesus Christ. I saw the ineffectiveness of a social movement such as the Black Panthers in changing a person's heart, and turned instead to the ultimate social activist, Jesus Christ, for answers. His message taught us to love our enemies, reach out to the poor and develop relationships with the marginalized—things that can only be done through the power of Christ in us.

In contrast, Birmingham, Alabama, was a city known at that time for racial and political violence. In the sixties the city was criticized for its segregation policies, police cruelty toward protesters and loss of innocent lives in the Sixteenth Street Baptist Church bombing. As with any social injustice, not everyone held biased views; there were many who embraced tolerance, love and acceptance. But the lines between blacks and whites seemed to be deeply drawn through the decades until they erupted during the civil rights movement. Much progress had been made in the years after the church bombing to bring the two groups together, but old attitudes remained in some ways on both sides. Faith and church life were extremely important in this southern city, but there was not much melding of the two cultures in churches.

This was the city I moved to in 1998 to be closer to my children, but I didn't feel like I belonged. People would say, "You're not from around here, are you?" I intentionally spoke in a precise manner, walked confidently into a room and held steady eye contact with others. I could also be outspoken and arrogant. I had been invited by a large white church to fill the role of urban ministry pastor, but that position only lasted three months because of differences in theology and political leanings. Our dissimilarities made it impossible for me to minister, so I left the job. (It is worth noting that the lead pastor, a godly man, helped me secure another job in the city.)

Because of this impasse, I retreated to a black church, but their style of preaching and worship was not part of my background either. I was stuck between two worlds. The distinctions between a "black church" and a "white church" were obvious in culture, political connections and generations of families. There seemed to be nothing in between. My wife and I went from one Birmingham church to another, trying to find our way. Where was a place of grace where we could land?

One weekday I was driving in Mountain Brook, a Birmingham suburb. Mountain Brook is the wealthiest city in Alabama and has been listed as one of America's most prosperous communities. More than 98 percent of the people in the city are white.[1] As I drove by the gracious homes on beautifully landscaped lots, I passed St. Peter's Anglican Church and was prompted by the Holy Spirit to go in. The pastor greeted me warmly and invited me into his study. He also assured me that I would be welcome in their fellowship. He explained that the small church of around two hundred members drew people from all over the metro area, as well as from other nations. He spoke of the worldwide Anglican community and its association with Rwanda and other African countries. I took him up on his offer and started visiting.

About two months later, he invited me to attend an Anglican convocation at the Birmingham Civic Center. I witnessed bishops from Uganda, Kenya, Rwanda, Tanzania, Mali and Nigeria filing down the aisles to join the American leadership. The Bishop of Rwanda spoke of the worldwide church as being unified, and he encouraged all bishops to be true to the gospel. I was amazed that this event was happening in Birmingham; the city that jailed Martin Luther King Jr. and resisted integrating blacks with whites was now receiving black bishops from Africa! And the little church I visited was connected to that larger community. After seeing this grace in action, I was compelled to become a part of it.

I had been a Christian Reformed pastor and church planter, but I wanted to become associated with the Anglican Church after watching the convocation. After a time of preparation and study, I was invited to travel to Rwanda for my ordination. African bishops ordained me into the priesthood and charged me to consider myself as a missionary to America.

When I returned to St. Peter's I was asked to be part of the pastoral care ministry and to participate in preaching. A few years later our church went through a leadership crisis that resulted in the pastor and some members leaving. Because of my disillusionment over the crisis, I also wanted to leave and asked our Rwandan bishop for permission to move on. He said, "No, Glandion, your witness as an African American priest in a predominantly white community is a powerful way for God to be glorified." He was prophetically correct, and I am grateful I stayed.

As I have continued at St. Peter's, I have experienced grace in community and ministered with a degree of love that I never thought possible. The stories that follow are examples of this.

LIFE TOGETHER

In the first chapter I wrote about disclosing my diagnosis of Parkinson's to the congregation. Since that time, the whole church body has rallied around me and shown grace in numerous and significant ways. For example, our new pastor moved my office from the second floor down to the first so that he can be next to me, ministering side by side and providing any needed assistance. This made it much easier physically to come and go. Several members of the church became my "decorating crew," choosing paint colors and coordinating furniture, tailoring the flow of the office to fit my needs.

With my disease comes an occasional "brain freeze" that immobilizes me; I cannot make a smooth transition from different surfaces like carpeting to tiled floors. My spiritual brothers and sisters are always there to give me a gentle push in the right direction or to turn me slightly in order to navigate a corner. Karen, the pastoral care deacon, drives on our visits to ailing parishioners, assisting me physically and spiritually. My cowriter, Marjean (who is also a member of our church), interprets my occasional faltering speech and makes my words flow beautifully. All of it is grace to me.

This fellowship of grace is also extended to the community at large as St. Peter's participates in a citywide ministry called Family Promise. Area churches unite to offer housing for families that are temporarily homeless, providing a place for them to stay in our church building for a week each quarter.[2] On one of these occasions, I went to have a meal with the guest families. A couple in their seventies brought dinner and served the meal, dishing out love and compassion with the meat and potatoes. A wealthy southern couple, they were gracious and genteel. I watched as the woman filled children's plates while her husband talked to a father. I can't describe exactly what I felt, but deep warmth and love for this couple came rushing into my heart. I have often referred to it as a "baptism of love."

Until that time, I had seen myself as a black priest associated with a white Anglican congregation. Even if they didn't see color, I did. The cultural and economic differences affected my ability to genuinely minister; I aimed to always be kind and considerate, yet I was guarded. But when I saw this couple loving a black family with such grace, my heart opened to them in a way that I can only describe as the feeling of falling in love. That experience laid the groundwork for me to live and serve honestly among this community. I allowed myself to be needy and open in the frailty of my disease, and in return I found I received more grace from others than I offered myself.

Because of this experience, I fully opened myself to be authentic with the entire church body. In return, they have opened up their lives with their struggles and failures. I learned that those who are rich in resources can also be poor in spirit. Those who *have* much can also *give* much, and many times I have been a recipient of their kindness. Money doesn't matter—it is an issue of the heart.

I have plenty of opportunity to participate in the giving and receiving of grace as the men at my church meet weekly in an early morning Bible study. I affectionately call them "the Grandfathers," and I credit this group for fostering a sense of community and belonging. In an era when women are known to be more open to things of the Spirit, it is encouraging to witness men growing and developing their spiritual lives, becoming vulnerable with one another. We all look forward to the meeting each week and encourage others to join us.

One man told me that what drew him to this group was open and honest sharing: "We voice our own thoughts and listen to what others have to say. Community is more important than any personal preferences, and we realize our differences are strengths. There are opposite ends of the spectrum present in personality and beliefs, but we still care about one another." Our group has experienced God's grace through relationship. We realize acceptance is a two-way street.

Although these are encouraging steps forward, our fellowship is not perfect and never will be. By God's grace, we are becoming more open and caring, willing to embrace each other and accept our differences. In fostering true community, the role of both receiving and extending grace cannot be underestimated.

THE GRACE OF COMMUNITY

As believers, there is a tendency to look to the church to meet our own needs. Many go from church to church just like I did, looking for the perfect one. But our search is futile—a perfect church does not exist this side of heaven. Bill White, a well-respected local counselor, said, "We have to realize that the presence and work of the Lord in community takes place in a fallen world, with fallen people who sin and are sinned against. To be a part of a life-giving community, you and I sometimes

have to lay aside some of what we want. Our personal preferences sometimes get in the way of what Christ is doing in the
lives of other people in the body."[3]

In some group settings there can still exist tinges of racism,
cultural elitism and self-importance. But this does not stop us from
desiring to be with one another, believing that God will overcome
our weaknesses and transform us. Developing close community is
like training to run a marathon—it takes patience, endurance and
strength. Change does not happen all at once. Spending time together through years of fellowship builds trust in relationship. We
crack the door and allow others to come in and see what we are
really like, which can eventually lead to sharing our lives on a
deeper level. Then the impact of God's grace moves into our fellowship; by acknowledging and sharing our own woundedness, we
can be healed and become a source of healing for others.

The book of Acts chronicles the formation and expansion of
the early church. Through the chapters, we see the apostle Paul
constantly ministering with a group of fellow workers. He only
traveled alone a few times; he was uncomfortable ministering to
others in isolation. In other words, he needed his team.

This mirrors what Jesus himself did. First, he exists in community in the mystery of the Godhead—Father, Son and Holy
Spirit, a triune God. Second, while on earth, he created a community of faith with the twelve disciples and a larger group of
followers, both men and women. This strategic unit became the
instrument of growth and expansion of the gospel, as people

were changed by Christ's message of grace and then shared it with others.

A third element is the forming of even smaller circles of intimacy. John, Peter and James were a type of "inner circle," chosen by Jesus to be part of some major events, such as the transfiguration and the raising of a little girl from the dead, and to be in closer presence to the Lord as he wept in the Garden of Gethsemane (Luke 9:18-36; Mark 5:35-43; Mark 14:32-34). In the same way, Paul and Barnabas ministered as a team for many years, and later the apostle mentored Timothy, calling him his son. A small group within a small group allows for deepening levels of intimacy, sharing life experiences and helping to bear one another's burdens. Grace in community lessens the load.

We can't effectively reach the world with the gospel without community. In what is known as the "high priestly prayer" recorded in John 17, Jesus said the world wouldn't believe the Father had sent him unless they witnessed unity in those who claimed to love him: "I in them and you in me, that they may become completely one, so that the world may know that you have sent me and have loved them even as you have loved me" (John 17:23). As difficult as it may be to understand, God uses sinful men and women in community with each other to show the world more about himself, his love and his grace.

THE SAFEST UNSAFE PLACE ON EARTH

In his book *The Safest Place on Earth*, Larry Crabb shares a vision of what the church should be—a loving community where each person is able to be open and vulnerable and, at the same time, be fully accepted and loved. Many have found the opposite to be true, which is tremendously sad. As one who tends to the wounds of others in spiritual direction, I have ministered to too many who have been rejected, hurt or judged by other believers in a time of need.

For example, one woman I knew was going to divorce her husband because he had been unfaithful and physically abusive. In spite of the danger she experienced at his hand, the church leadership insisted she stay with her husband or lose the privilege of being a part of the church. Eventually she found safety and lived under a different name. After sharing a burden with her pastor and leadership, this woman suffered greatly when they showed no grace for her physical and emotional welfare.

Many others have been wounded by a lack of love or concern for their needs. When they have needed a loving touch or an encouraging word, the church has not been the grace-filled place to find it. Many have been judged when they have opened up about a prevailing sin in their lives. Others have been criticized for their lack of faith. In one church, when a woman died from cancer despite receiving healing prayers from others, her family was told she did not have enough faith to get well.

Grace—or the lack of it—is a huge issue. Scripture encourages transparency and honesty with other believers, but many people struggle to respond well to openness, brokenness and vulnerability. Some don't know how to hold confidences well. Others have not dealt with their own woundedness, so they withdraw in fear or respond in a judgmental and accusatory manner to those who are brave enough to open up.

In contrast, I have also witnessed great caring and love by the body of Christ for its members, as in the story of my friend Chollet. While in her fifties, Chollet was diagnosed with breast cancer and underwent chemotherapy and radiation. Her immediate family, as well as our church family, gathered around her like a human shield and ministered to her in this time of great need. Our pastoral care deacon, Karen, and I went to her home often to surround her with healing prayers. She said, "When I was diagnosed with cancer, the community of grace was here waiting for me. I felt like all I had to do was show up and receive." She experienced beautiful touches of compassion as others brought meals, sent cards and ran errands while she was down. Because of these loving actions by so many, Chollet said she felt as if God had sent his angels to care for her.

This time of both sickness and received grace changed Chollet in many ways. It made her more comfortable with other people's illnesses. Where before she might have hesitated to visit someone who was ill, now she is quick to go. She offers to accompany others to their chemotherapy appointments and helps women pick out wigs when they reach the difficult stage of losing their hair. She is quicker to do for others what has been done for her. Chollet is known to say, "I have cancer. Cancer doesn't have me. This disease is part of the journey, but it doesn't define who I am. Others helped me to see this."

That is the beauty of grace-filled community—Jesus showing up in the midst of wounded people, healing them and sending them out to minister to others. They become, then, a fellowship of wounded healers. This describes what Dietrich Bonhoeffer, German theologian and martyr, meant when he penned the phrase "sacramental community."

I started this chapter with the question of what I had in common with other believers of different color and culture in the South. I thought it was nothing, but instead I have found it is everything. There is no difference in our hearts, needs or humanity. We are the same. As Jesus touches each of us with his grace, we in turn touch each other. In that way, we are all wounded healers.

REFLECTION

The challenges to building community are great, but I believe there are three major components that can help to accomplish a spirit of grace within a body of believers:

1. *Deep conviction about corporate Christianity.* It is not just about our own relationship with God but also the profound value of the fellowship of believers. Yes, we are individual in our relationship with God, but we are woven together in community, making us stronger and more effective in our

faith. There is no "lone wolf" theology found in Scripture; in fact, there are fifty-nine "one another" verses listed in the New Testament. "Be at peace with one another" (Mark 9:50), "Love one another" (John 15:17) and "Be devoted to one another in brotherly love" (Romans 12:10 NASB) are just a few.

2. *Knowing and being known.* This requires spending time together. Hopefully, after coming to know one another more intimately, each person grows in his or her willingness to be open and honest, which paves the community highway. This step encourages us to embrace our woundedness, which is sometimes the hardest thing to do. It is easier to find the faults of others and to spend time criticizing them. But it can be very freeing to realize that none of us has it all together. The more we embrace that worldview, the more we see others through the lens of grace and less through the lens of critique.

3. *Gospel-grace orientation.* A deep conviction that we are all sinners breaks down any superiority issues and keeps us from judging. As Jesus said, "Why do you see the speck in your neighbor's eye, but do not notice the log in your own eye?" (Matthew 7:3). Gospel-grace orientation reminds us that we are all in this together; we are broken and needy people who come to God for healing and restoration. Grace also calls us to forgive, which can be one of the biggest tests we face. Part of

the answer is to pray for the person who has offended us, as a major part of Christian fellowship is praying and interceding for one another. We become burden bearers for one another.

In doing this, we take stock of our calling and realize that God has given us a gift that is necessary to the body of believers. It is up to us whether or not we choose to share it. It is our task to weave the components of knowing and being known, gospel-grace orientation, and a conviction about the value of corporate Christianity together in order to have a viable opportunity of true fellowship and a community motivated by grace.

APPLICATION

Are you struggling to enter into the grace of community with others? These questions might be helpful in determining what is blocking fellowship:

- What judgments or prejudices are stopping you from entering into deep relationship with others?

- Are you allowing a hidden sin, bitterness or an illness to dictate whether you are finding meaning and a place in church?

- Do you find it easy to withdraw from others because of the hurt in your life?

- Are you looking for the "perfect" church before you show grace to others and enter into fellowship? Be open to experience community on a deeper level right where you are before seeking a new environment.

Bring any of these things to our Father in confession and prayer.

Father, forgive me for withdrawing from both you and the community of faith at times. Give me the grace to be an open and willing part of the fellowship of the saints. Please take the log out of my own eye so that I might see clearly to tend to the needs of others. Amen.

A Cup of Cool Water

The Grace of Comfort

Insomnia.

Sleeplessness is one of Parkinson's most debilitating effects. It's nothing for me to wake at three and be up for the rest of the day. I find that I do my deepest thinking in these early morning hours. It is the most honest part of my day, when reality sinks in as I reflect on life, death, past sorrows, hopes and fears. I am taken to the edge and back again. Things like despair and wondering what has meaning or purpose send me on an existential quest. I usually don't find it to be a time of great comfort from God; instead I feel like he ponders with me, saying, "We'll think together." I relate to Job in Scripture when he utters, "I go about in sunless gloom; I stand up in the assembly and cry for help" (Job 30:28).

In these predawn hours, I contemplate what it means to be a

disciple of Jesus. I spend time thinking about how to love my wife and minister to her in a Christ-honoring way. My illness-driven moodiness, which I experience daily, seems to affect everything. At times my petty differences with Marion seem to loom large. I have become defensive about her desire to help me eat healthily and her concern about my rest or inconsistency with medication.

I feel I have lost control of my life, and this is especially devastating at home. I struggle with the fact that, out of necessity, Marion must be in charge, calling the doctor, reminding me not to carry too much up the stairs, instructing me how to care for my cell phone. In order to cope, I often become passive-aggressive. I stuff the feelings down, but they seep out in defiant behavior.

I have a debilitating illness. In many areas, I have lost the option of doing what I want. It's difficult and humbling, and can make me angry. I am mad at the circumstances, but instead I lash out at those who love me the most.

When I sit and contemplate in the early morning hours, the bigger realities humble me—life is short, I could die, and I must live by grace. This is the moment I'm tempted to believe the lie that I have to earn grace by "doing it right." It is during this time that I repent most authentically, crying out to God and receiving the strength to carry on. I want to live and serve well, but as the day progresses, it's more and more of a challenge.

Marion wants to be known as my wife, not a caregiver. But in reality, she is both. Marriage is more than caring for another;

it is a lifelong three-strand partnership between you, your spouse and God. Part of the wedding vow is to be faithful to the end, in sickness and in health. In doing this for me, Marion provides the grace of comfort. She has become "Jesus with skin on," and for that, I am grateful.

When you are in pain it is not always easy to recognize comfort. And it often changes the nature of relationships. I want to make sure, while I am still able, to address some of the feelings that have arisen around the issue of pain and the provision of comfort. I am attempting to be as open and honest as possible. Although some thoughts are almost too painful to record, it is my hope that these words will speak to someone who desperately needs to hear them.

SHARING THE PAIN

At one of his last concerts, world-famous guitarist Jimi Hendrix is reported to have said, "What is truth? Does anyone know what truth is?" It's a question that has haunted me in different areas of my life for many years. This chapter is an attempt to tell the truth about where I am and how I see pain affecting my dearest relationships. Disease does not only affect the one who is ill; it touches all who are in close relationship with the patient, especially the family members.

In many moments of my life I have not been a model husband or father and have put work before my family. I have shown concern for others and had none left for those at home. But, time and time again, I've asked forgiveness, and in the past I felt I was strong enough to fix things in my own power. Now things are changing and I can't pull it off anymore. Maybe I never could and my sense of control was only an illusion.

What's changed?

I fear I'm no longer the physically strong man my wife married or the approachable father my children ran to for support. I cry easily. I often withdraw into my own mind, attempting to find respite from depression over the effects of Parkinson's. I spend much of my time being introspective in a quiet room. My doctor says this is a part of the disease, but in many ways it is a new chapter for me. Increasingly I find myself wanting to ask those closest to me, "Can we hold off talking about the bad parts of our day and just be still and quiet together?" But I fear I will hurt them with that question.

Many things bother me. I'm sad that I can't serve my family by fixing a meal like I used to. I'm frustrated by how long it takes me to do simple chores. I'm embarrassed that, because of a weak bladder, I make a mess in the bathroom. Before I can clean it up, others are there to do it for me.

I am consumed with moodiness and preoccupied with symptoms. I seem to get all the attention from those around us, while my wife is in the background. I find myself thinking about other things instead of listening as she talks to me about her concerns. We have said we would grow old together, and yet I feel I am outpacing her. This frightens me and seems greatly unfair. I grieve about having a disease that is robbing us of the adventures we had planned for this time in our lives.

It bothers me that my wife has had to take over the majority of the driving and other daily tasks like bringing in groceries, fixing things around the house and writing my correspondence. I am grateful she does these things, but I'm not sure how well I communicate that sentiment to her. It has become hard for me to express myself and enter into everyday life; either I'm lost in contemplation or I'm too tired to try.

Although I would like to suggest that my family and I pray and have devotions together, I find it easier to do them alone. But when I do struggle through and initiate times of spiritual togetherness, I find it always draws us closer.

I know that others, especially Marion, are serving me out of love. But I also realize it comes at great cost, as those who care for a Parkinson's patient are often taxed. I see the fatigue etched on her face. I know my family worries about many things. How will the illness progress? How will the next step change things? What's around the corner? I realize these concerns take energy and creativity away from them, vitality they would normally devote to other people and pursuits.

Many say, "You're doing too much." I explain that I need to do much, because it proves I'm still living. Not to do much would make me feel like I am losing the battle and Parkinson's is winning. I know they are trying to protect me, but I have to do these things now while I still have the energy and will to do them. They say, "You are seeing too many people." But I want to meet with people while I can.

My family worries about me as I pray for others and carry their burdens. Yet I consider it a privilege to do this for those who trust me with their concerns. As a result, those closest to me often feel that I don't carry their burdens. I am trying to be aware of this and to make a conscious effort to be there for my loved ones.

I'm grateful for my work, which allows me to be independent in some ways. As a pastor, I too have a life of service. Providing care to my congregation gives me a feeling of worth and helps me feel useful.

I'm also grateful for other things I can still do, like playing with my grandkids. I am happy that I'm able to call our children once a week and be part of their lives. It is a blessing that they allow me to be honest with them about my progression or regression and to share in their problems as well.

In one of my favorite pictures, Marion and I are sitting on a boat listening to jazz. I'm in white, rolled-up pants and sunglasses, with my Kangol hat on backwards. We each have a glass of wine in our hands, and my arm rests around her shoulders. She is smiling playfully as the breeze blows her hair. To me this photo portrays the ultimate joy in being satisfied with life, and Marion is there by my side.

I'm grateful for many things, like the vacations my wife and I have had in the past, the long hikes in the mountains and adventures in San Francisco. I treasure her faithfulness, her consistently steady spirit and her support in helping me make wise health choices. It's an encouragement when she organizes my office. I appreciate that she works hard in her job, and then comes home to another. She's patient with me when I wake in the night and loves me even when I do not love her well.

In the next few months we'll decide whether I should have deep brain stimulation. That sounds ominous to all of us. In this procedure, an implant will be placed in my brain to stop the advancing symptoms of Parkinson's. Along with other tests, one requirement is a four-hour interview with a psychologist and a neurologist. Another step in this procedure is having your spouse involved in the decision-making process. I can only imagine how hard it must be for Marion to help me decide whether to have surgery when the results are so risky. We know this operation could help reduce my symptoms, have little effect or, in rare cases, cause death.

So now, while I can, I want to publicly thank Marion for being my lover, supporter, cheerleader and burden bearer, as well as my friend. I am glad that at six in the morning when she stirs, I can bring her coffee in bed and say, "Good morning."

She has been caring, loving and forgiving, and at times, tough. After forty-five years, it is a blessing that we are still celebrating life together. I am grateful she has been there through it all. I can never thank her enough for providing God's comfort to me.

THE GRACE OF COMFORT

Receiving comfort in the grace of God is not always a feeling or an emotional high. It is a deep sense of knowing that God is faithful while learning to be alone and quiet with him. We cannot create this grace for ourselves; it is a gift. It is God-given and helps us face life honestly. God is always near and ready to offer consolation. Without his tender mercies we are left to our own thoughts, which can be accusing or shameful. Comfort humbles us because we can't produce it ourselves; we must depend on God to supply it. The beauty of this provision is shown in 1 Peter 5:5, "God . . . gives grace to the humble."

In addition to receiving comfort from my wife and family, I've also learned to draw consolation from God throughout the day. I often sit in his presence with a cup of coffee, reading Scripture or listening to music. The song "10,000 Reasons" by Matt Redman is especially meaningful to me. He encourages me, from Psalm 103, to "Bless the LORD, O my soul, and all that is within me, bless his holy name," as it is possible to find ten thousand reasons for our hearts to praise him. I try to remember to praise him for the blessings I *do* have, even as I pour out my soul before him for what I *don't* have. As I list my difficulties and requests, I also list the reasons I have to be grateful. One major blessing is that I feel safe in my relationship with God, knowing he loves me no matter what.

In Scripture many received the grace of comfort. One of Joseph's sons, Ephraim, encountered a tragedy when his four sons were killed in battle. First Chronicles 7:22 says, "And their father Ephraim mourned many days, and his brothers came to comfort him." In this example, comfort was found in a human touch. But the divine touch is also evident in Scripture. In Isaiah 40:1 we read, "Comfort, O comfort my people, says your God." Later in Isaiah 51:12 he reveals, "I am he who comforts you." We can know him as *the God of all comfort*.

In Genesis 16, God showed up in a tender way in the story of Hagar, who was Abraham and Sarah's handmaid. Since the couple had produced no heir and were advanced in age, Sarah tried to remedy the problem by giving her servant to Abraham in order to have a child. But this "quick fix" backfired. Sarah treated Hagar harshly when she got pregnant, and Hagar despised her mistress. Eventually Hagar fled. The angel of the Lord appeared to Hagar and gave reassurances regarding Ishmael, the child she was carrying. In this passage we see God's amazing concern for a woman who was simply a servant. It was to Hagar that the angel revealed one of God's names: *El-roi*, the God who sees. This story paints the picture of a God who sees our pain and interacts with us in the midst of it, no matter who we are or our station in life. He sees, and he cares.

David was the master of turning to God, pouring out his soul and receiving comfort from on high. In more than eighty Psalms penned by David, he recorded every emotion known to man— anguish, joy, loneliness, anger, fear, depression, confidence, despair, hopelessness, jealousy and feelings of betrayal. He too suffered the effects of sleeplessness. But he never gave up, no matter how difficult his circumstances. He comforted himself in the Lord, and in the most famous Psalm of all, recorded the timeless line that has consoled believers through the ages: "Even though I walk through the valley of the shadow of death, I fear no evil, for You are with me; Your rod and Your staff, they comfort me" (Psalm 23:4 NASB).

Jesus had much to say about comfort. He stated that his coming fulfilled the Old Testament prophecy in Isaiah 61:1-3, "The Spirit of the Lord GOD is upon me . . . *to comfort all who mourn*; to provide for those who mourn in Zion—to give them a garland instead of ashes, the oil of gladness instead of mourning" (emphasis added). He told his disciples that part of the fulfillment of this comfort was God sending the Holy Spirit, *the Comforter*, to indwell all believers (John 14:16). We have a built-in source of comfort to draw from when we are struggling; he is as close as our breath. Indeed, the Hebrew word for Spirit, *ruah*, actually means "breath."

The early church learned to draw from God's strength, for we read in Acts 9:31 that "the church throughout Judea, Galilee, and Samaria had peace and was built up. Living in the fear of the Lord and in the comfort of the Holy Spirit, it increased in numbers." Jesus also promised to return one day, ushering in the kingdom of God. In 1 Thessalonians 4:18, Paul says to "comfort one another with these words" (NASB) regarding the second coming.

As we receive comfort from God, we are able to comfort

others. In 2 Corinthians 1:3-4, we read that the "God of all comfort . . . comforts us in all our affliction so that we may be able to comfort those who are in any affliction with the comfort with which we ourselves are comforted by God" (NASB). In God's economy, nothing is wasted. God comforts us, not so we are comfortable, but so that we may become comforters ourselves.

THE LEAST OF THESE

Our journey starts when we realize our own poverty and neediness. We come to God for comfort in all our afflictions. Then, as we receive comfort from God, we seek to provide the same for others. But I'll be honest with you, this is a daily battle— there is no "storing up of comfort" for the next day. Just like drinking a cup of cool water, we cannot drink enough in one day to supply the need for the next. Daily drinking at his well is needed through prayer, Scripture and meditation on God.

Mother Teresa was a shining example of the grace of comfort, and volumes have been written about her life and ministry. As a Catholic nun, she left the comfort of the convent to serve "the poorest of the poor" on the streets of Calcutta, India. She began the Missionaries of Charity, an order of women who gave up all that they owned to identify with those who had nothing. They sought to bring relief to the sick and dying, considering these unfortunate ones the same as their Lord who suffered and said, "I thirst."

This example challenges us to follow in their footsteps, reaching out to others with love and comfort. Mother Teresa said, "We can do no great things—only small things done with great love."[1] Surely she must have received a double portion of the grace of comfort herself, enabling her to pour out to so many.

Mother Teresa also stressed the importance of silence. She said that prayer was not as much talking to God as it was listening for his voice. In silence, we hear and connect, receiving his comfort. This eventually leads to comforting others. Her five guiding principles for life show the progression: "The fruit of silence is prayer. The fruit of prayer is faith. The fruit of faith is love. The fruit of love is service. The fruit of service is peace."[2]

REFLECTION

Not everyone can take a vow of poverty and devote him- or herself to meeting the needs of the poor. But the examples of others can encourage us to become aware of how we might provide comfort to those around us.

Many times when I am eating out, I take time to notice the waiter's face or posture. I ask how I can pray for him or her, which usually brings an open and honest response. The server often takes risks to tell me deep things—struggles with breast cancer, or a brain tumor, or simply the desire to get away to go fishing. I don't pray with the server right then unless specifically asked to do so. But later on I lift up the request to God. It's interesting to see how much it means to a stranger when I take the time to notice and acknowledge his or her need, or simply address that person by name.

Jesus used three forms of comfort with his disciples on the road to Emmaus in Luke 24. First, he joined them in their *conversation*. He can join us in conversation personally, as well as with others. Second, he enlightened them with the *Scriptures,* opening both their minds and eyes to recognize his presence among them. And third, he *broke bread* with them in fellowship around a meal. These are simple, interpersonal touches that revealed his concern, care and comfort.

If the God of the universe has time to come into the lives of his children by walking with, eating with and listening to them, we can make time for others too. We can bring comfort simply by choosing to enter their world. John Stott said, "Grace is love that cares and stoops and rescues."[3] The comfort you give doesn't have to have an awe factor. It can be simple and honest. It is up to us to take the time to consider another's needs and make the decision to follow in Christ's steps by ministering to those around us.

APPLICATION

Let Jesus join you in conversation. In your devotions, read through a Gospel (Matthew, Mark, Luke or John) and notice how Jesus offered comfort in the most practical ways—a touch, a word or a walk with his friends.

Music, especially spiritual music, can be a powerful source of comfort as different songs minister to your soul. Take time to listen, opening your heart to receive comfort from the Holy Spirit.

Participating in communion can be a means of comfort as you "break bread" with Jesus and other believers.

Comfort yourself (and others) with the words of 2 Thessalonians 2:16-17:

"Now may our Lord Jesus Christ himself and God our Father, who loved us and through grace gave us eternal comfort and good hope, comfort your hearts and strengthen them in every good work and word."

LIFE IN THE SLOW LANE

The Grace of Simplicity

MY MORNING ROUTINE IS SIMPLE: Get up, drink coffee, take a shower and get dressed. I've repeated this pattern thousands of times over forty years without any problem. But one morning as I put on my shirt, my fingers couldn't grasp the buttons and push them through the holes. I thought to myself, "Hmmm, too much starch." I tried another shirt, then another and another, trying to find one that was not so stiff. There was a stack of discarded shirts as high as Mt. Everest before I found one I could conquer.

My first response was to let it go and not worry about it. I would tell the dry cleaners not to use so much starch! But when this dilemma happened again the next day, and the next, not being able to push a button through a hole convinced me this was not an easy fix. I was angry. What was going on with me?

Why couldn't I do something so simple? Suddenly a simple task I learned as a child was daunting, insurmountable. Instead of a mindless step in getting ready for the day, buttoning a shirt became a burdensome task that required my full attention.

This frustration went on for about a month with the same results, always ending in anger. The process of pushing a button through a hole should not lead to rage. Some days I would stop midshirt, leave the rest of the buttons undone and throw on a sports coat or sweater to cover my failure.

In defeat I asked Marion to button my shirts. She was glad to help, and it only took her a minute to do this. Accepting assistance for something I was used to doing for myself helped me calm down. I relinquished this duty to her instead of raging over the futility.

Gradually I asked God for the grace to button my shirt without being uptight. When Marion wasn't there to do it for me, I attempted the task again with a new attitude. I called it "my little experiment," and each button became an extension of the Lord's Prayer (see Matthew 6:9-13). While working on the first button, I focused on "Our Father," and contemplated the love God has for me. God became my friend, one who was helping me with a task. This simple two-word prayer allowed me to slow down and breathe, continuing to work the button while concentrating on God. In about ten minutes, I moved to the second one. "Hallowed be your name" prompted me to meditate on the beauty of God's names and the comfort they brought—Abba "Daddy," Adonai "Lord," and Yahweh "the self-sufficient One." On the third button I recited, "Your kingdom come," and continued through each phrase until the task was accomplished. The process usually took an hour of concentrated work, and prayer, to finish successfully.

Instead of inciting anger, this exercise allowed me to begin my day slowly and with worship. I hid spiritual truths in my heart as I concentrated on prayerful words instead of a maddening task. It also prepared me for my appointments with others during the course of the day, as I encouraged them to claim God's love and fatherhood in their own lives. Insights from my experiment provided a great "Aha!" moment for me to share with other people that related to their own issues—whether it was frustration while driving in traffic, dealing with difficult people, complex personal issues or sitting in endless meetings.

Focusing on simplicity transformed the mundane into a sacrament. I knew it was a gift of God's grace to bring me to this point, as this patient practice was not something I would naturally do. If I could be changed in this way, so could anyone.

Driving was another challenge. When I first got sick with Parkinson's, friends would see me driving slowly around town and report this to my family. I thought slower, therefore I drove slower, and the fact that other cars were moving at such a rapid speed made me panic. Other drivers became irate as they attempted to go around me. Their reaction is a symbol of our fast-paced way of life; everyone appears to be on his or her own mission with speed being one of the requirements. Indeed, the whole adventure in slowing down is countercultural—everyone else is speeding up, navigating the fast lane. It seems there is no such thing as a slow lane anymore. Eventually I had to give up driving and depend on others to take me where I needed to go.

I've also developed a stutter because of my illness, and it takes me longer to get my words out. I saw no grace in *that* at all. But there is one—I look for simple words to express myself now, one or two syllables to convey thought. I'm finding the grace to be content in this as well.

At first I resented the move to simplicity and slowing down. But without other options, I learned to tolerate it. Gradually I learned to embrace it. The grace of simplicity actually worked for my benefit as it taught me the importance of calming myself, contemplating truth and living with a sense of purpose.

THE GRACE OF SIMPLICITY

With the onset of Parkinson's, my schooling in simplicity became more like an advanced-degree course. I was a novice, at best, on this subject, and I had difficulty implementing the practice in a busy life. But as I experienced and cultivated simplicity in unexpected areas, it became a grace—God's love flowing to me in the midst of difficulties. It enabled me to focus on what is truly important, much like a kaleidoscope of jumbled fragments that suddenly sharpens into a lovely design.

The grace of simplicity has been well documented by

Christian saints through the ages who are noted for their exquisite writings: Brother Lawrence, Bishop Fenelon, James Bryan Smith, Richard Foster and others. These writers captured the beauty of simplicity, as found in Fenelon's quote:

> When we are truly in this interior simplicity our whole appearance is franker, more natural. This true simplicity . . . makes us conscious of a certain openness, gentleness, innocence, gaiety, and serenity, which is charming when we see it near to and continually, with pure eyes. O, how amiable this simplicity is! Who will give it to me? I leave all for this. It is the Pearl of the Gospel.[1]

On my desk is a sculpture of an ancient Chinese man sitting on a stone. His hand is extended in front of him, holding a nail-scarred cross. He is bent in concentration, with eyes fixed on the cross. It is a reminder of the quote from the classic Chinese text *Tao Te Ching*, "Be content in what you have. Rejoice in the way things are. When you realize there is nothing lacking, the whole world belongs to you."[2] As I look at the sculpture I sense the man's inner peace, and it challenges me to focus on what matters most. When I take the time to simplify my thoughts, I look differently at my circumstances. I also view others in a changed way—recognizing each has his or her unique set of needs and issues.

I valued many things prior to my move toward simplicity: multitasking, being with one person yet thinking about the person to come afterward, packing my schedule with as many tasks as I could, checking them off with pride and planning a full schedule for the following day. These are not bad things, but this simple grace has allowed me to pause, take life more slowly and listen to every word as someone speaks. I agree with Richard Foster's statement that simplicity is freedom; it brings joy and balance to our lives. The grace of simplicity becomes an inward reality that results in a different outward lifestyle.[3]

We counter the common way of the modern world—which is always adding more and more—by intentionally using or having less. Less food. Less energy. Less stuff. When we are not focused on material accumulation and ourselves, we paradoxically have more to give to others. It becomes a means toward the holy end of spiritual transformation. If we simplify our lives as an end in itself, the process can become drudgery. We must allow the grace of simplicity to energize and expand our ability to nurture our own souls and reach out to nurture others. Out of this grace comes a deeper contentment and gratitude for what we have: health, friends, food, clothing, heat in winter, cool air in summer, family and shelter.[4]

SAINTS OF SIMPLICITY

Brother Lawrence was a monk who lived in the 1400s. His little book *The Practice of the Presence of Jesus* grew out of letters he wrote to an unknown recipient. In these writings, he reveals the secret of communing with Jesus on a moment-by-moment basis. His was a practice of simplicity mixed with thankfulness. As he worked in the monastery's kitchen, he was aware of God's presence even in the simple act of washing a pot. He taught the value of being conscious of ordinary things that become quite beautiful when noticed: the feel of warm dishwater, the exquisite beauty of a single bloom, the aroma of fresh-baked bread. He encourages us to notice and appreciate the moment, but we have to train ourselves to slow down, recognize and value it.

Jesus is described in the Bible as a man who lived simply while on earth. He wore only ordinary tunics and sandals, and he had "nowhere to lay his head" (Matthew 8:20). He was driven by a singular goal—"My food is to do the will of him who sent me and to complete his work" (John 4:34). He lived the ultimate life of simplicity while fulfilling the grandest of all missions. We see him fully present in each moment, situation and encounter with another person. He lived simply yet powerfully and fulfilled his purpose that others might simply live. He came that we "may have life, and have it abundantly" (John 10:10).

Other Scriptures teach about the grace of simplicity. The book of Proverbs exhorts, "Better is a little with the fear of the LORD, than great treasure and trouble with it" (Proverbs 15:16). When the Pharisees asked Jesus which was the greatest commandment, he boiled down the entire Law with a simple answer that held profound implications: "'You shall love the Lord your God with all your heart, and with all your soul, and with all your mind.' This is the greatest and first commandment. And a second is like it: 'You shall love your neighbor as yourself'" (Matthew

22:37-39). The apostle Paul points to the disciples' simple message and manner when he says in 2 Corinthians 1:12, "Indeed, this is our boast, the testimony of our conscience: we have behaved in the world with frankness and godly sincerity, not by earthly wisdom but by the grace of God—and all the more toward you."

Simplicity purifies a relationship and reveals beauty. It heightens the act of looking into another's eyes, listening to the familiarity of a voice or sharing contented times of silence. This relates to our time spent with God as well. It is humbling to realize that all you have to offer God is your mind, your life and your soul; "Nothing in my hands I bring, simply to the cross I cling."[5] He, in turn, offers his grace back to you to help sanctify these offerings. It is simple, yet profound.

'TIS A GIFT TO BE SIMPLE, TO BE FREE

Recently I visited with a fellow priest and counselor, Don Richards. We discussed the subject of simplicity in life and vocation. He finds the grace of simplicity crucial to ministering in the Spirit, as his days are filled to overflowing with the struggles of others. When confronted with his clients' complicated issues, he seeks to speak only the words Jesus would speak and do only the things Jesus would do. He maintains an attitude of continual prayer as he listens.

In his personal life, Don gets away from a stressful world by retreating outdoors for long periods of time, including a yearly backpacking trip with his wife in the mountains of the western

United States. Those three weeks are like water to his parched soul. They usually walk more than one hundred miles and sleep in a little tent for weeks at a time. The beauty of the Lord's creation often brings them to their knees.

Don also participates in a yearly ministry trip to Africa, where the Maasai have taught him powerful lessons about simplicity. (The Maasai are an ethnic group of seminomadic people located in Kenya and northern Tanzania.) He told me that he gets dirty and stays dirty. It's okay with him—he likes it and is getting accustomed to his own smell. He is only concerned with basic things like dirt; a nose full of red dust, sweat and water; and rice for three meals a day, seven days a week. He values a hat that hasn't been washed in six years. He likes walking, straining, being exhausted and accomplishing simple physical effort. This is his story:

The Kenyan Maasai took me into the bush for three days. My idea of simplicity was a small backpack, a small tent and a small sleeping bag. The native men took a stick, a spear and a shuka (a simple, thin blanket). They didn't take water, food or means for lighting a fire. They found water, they found food, and they made fire from sticks. They found Kudu dung and placed the ember in the dung for a fire, where they roasted some kind of animal they killed. They drank the water in muddy puddles, which was thick and rancid. I'll never forget getting up in the morning and looking over at them wrapped in their shukas, watching the sun come up.

Besides their simplistic resourcefulness, the way they face death is striking. Since there are no funeral homes or morticians, the Maasai are not able to separate themselves from the realities of death and dying because they are close. They face death with unbelievable acceptance—I saw a kind of a joy that I almost never see associated with it here. The week before my arrival, my friend Charles lost his brother in a motorcycle accident about five hundred yards from the village. His brother was in his thirties, married with two young children. Charles built his brother's casket, dug his grave, laid him in the casket and covered him with the earth. There were tears of sorrow, but these were mixed with tears of joyous expectation. He knew he would see him again one day.

I witnessed their simplicity in celebration, too. On one of my trips, a man's prize cow had died the day I arrived. It was an occasion to have a bunch of folks come over to help butcher it. I shared in both butchering and eating the bounty. Along with the meat, they had rice, beans, water and goat's milk.

Simplistic grace is also extended to those who are physically challenged; in the Maasai culture, being physically or mentally challenged makes these individuals special and elevates their position. Instead of feeling sorry for them, they think, "Whoa, God must love them a lot."

It's funny how we in the Western world feel our complicated and fast-paced lives are superior to those in third-world coun-

tries. The Maasai have shown me the grace of simplicity in ways I would have never seen at home. God gives this grace to those who are humble and willing to receive.

SUBTRACTION, NOT ADDITION

Basic math can be used to picture simplicity. Grace doesn't flow by *adding* more and more to our lives; instead it fills the places where we have *subtracted* extraneous elements. In the article "Simply Focused: Uncluttering the Christian Life," Chris Tiegreen writes:

> For much of my life, I've made the Christian life more difficult than it really is—kind of like doing all sorts of mental gymnastics to solve a detailed math problem when the only essential detail is in the first phrase. It isn't that there aren't details to factor in or deeper truths we can learn or other angles to consider. But any spiritual instruction that takes us away from gazing *at* Christ rather than *toward* him is not helpful.[6]

Simplicity and purpose come from spending quiet times gazing intently at Jesus, not just distractedly looking his way while moving on with life. World-renowned performance consultant, motivational speaker and author Kevin Elko adds,

> If a person wants more peace, that person does not need to add anything. Instead, that person must rid himself of

whatever is not "peace"; then, more peace will find that person. Would you like a better marriage? Are you and your spouse doing something that wrongly impacts your marriage? Get rid of it, and a good marriage will find you. Sometimes, if you simply focus on letting go of needing to be right, whispering to yourself, "I must let go of my insistence," you will be just about there. Surprisingly, you don't even need to find God! *Rid your life of what is not God, and He will find you.*[7]

REFLECTION

I remember one Fourth of July when a steady rain fell all day long. A severe weather system had set in for several days, calming all the usual activities surrounding the holiday weekend. Instead of being active outdoors, entertained by bands, parades and fireworks, everyone was inside. The rain had washed away all the distractions.

The grace of simplicity does the same thing in our interior lives. When we get away from all the "do's" of the Christian life, we find the heart of devotion and worship in simple things—gazing at Christ, loving him, falling at his feet, asking him what is on his mind instead of informing him of what is on ours. We learn to see beauty in subtraction instead of concentrating on addition. We slow down to accomplish a task instead of raging at our helplessness. And the end result is grace—God's gift of simplicity flowing down to wash out the debris in our lives.

It is much like a pruning process, the cleaning out of unnecessary branches that are inhibiting growth of fruit. We can choose to do this ourselves in order to blossom, or the Lord will do it for us, for "He removes every branch in me that bears no fruit. Every branch that bears fruit he prunes to make it bear more fruit" (John 15:2).

Are you confident in your ability to prune the branches yourself? If not, ask our Father to bring out the shears, and he will gladly do this for you. Ask God for the grace to simplify your life.

APPLICATION

What aspects of simplicity resonate with your spirit? Where do you need to make changes? Don't try to do this all at once—just being aware of the need to begin is the first step. Try one simple adjustment each day.

You might begin the day slowly, resisting the urge to check your email or scroll through the endless possibilities on your phone. Sit quietly for five minutes and breathe. Concentrate on the stillness, the sound of a bird or the hum of a fan. Use a simple prayer to recite daily, paying attention to each word and saying it slowly.

Father, I ask for the grace of simplicity in my life today. Please teach me how to live and how to love others. Give me the ability to subtract rather than add. Amen.

A Shaker song also encourages us to embrace simplicity in our lives.

'Tis the gift to be simple,
  'tis the gift to be free,
'Tis the gift to come down
  where we ought to be,
And when we find ourselves in the place just right,
  'twill be in the valley of love and delight.
When true simplicity is gained
  to bow and to bend we shan't be ashamed,
  to turn, turn, will be our delight
Till by turning, turning we come 'round right.
—"Simple Gifts"

9

Possibilities

The Grace of Hope

✍

I was on the operating table, waiting for deep brain stimulation. The nurses prepped and shaved me, and gave me some "woozy juice" to sedate me. Then they placed a metal basket-looking device over my head and tightened four screws to hold it in place. In my drugged state, I kept thinking, "Drill, baby, drill."

After months of preparation, I was ready. Fear had been conquered, and the future was bright. I was awake to respond to commands and aid in the proper insertion of the probes, but thankfully anesthesia controlled the pain.

The doctors were encouraging; they felt this operation would alter my Parkinson's symptoms and reduce the need for more medication. They also felt it would increase my energy and movement, and help regulate my moods a little better. As I struggled to get through a doorway during those last few weeks before surgery, I'd tell others, "Soon I'll have surgery to take care of this!" When I dozed off in a conversation, I'd wake up and say, "With the new stimulator, I'll be more alert." I had great expectations, and hope was flying high.

The lights in the operating room were intense. Suddenly a shadow fell over my eyes as the lead doctor bent down and said, "Glandion, I don't feel good about this surgery today. I don't care what the tests say—I don't have a good feeling about it." My blood had been tested seven or eight times, and one of the last tests raised a concern that it might not coagulate correctly. They were even more cautious than usual because I had been taking a blood thinner due to another condition.

Suddenly the surgery was off. They removed all the paraphernalia and shut down the machines. I laid on the table in disbelief. My hopes were demolished. Why would God put such hopefulness in front of me only to have it disappear like a snowflake landing in a hot fire?

I spent the next week in the hospital being tested for every possible disease—cancer, HIV and rare blood conditions. No one knew why my blood levels were off, and the answers didn't come right away. While I waited in my private room, interns came in to say, "Stay hopeful." But I felt far from hopeful. Messages from the Holy Spirit kept coming to me through the hospital chaplain, nurses who cared and friends who prayed over me. Everyone tried to buoy my spirits.

Researchers studying my case called experts around the country as they tried to figure out what was happening and why. They finally concluded the irregular blood test results must have been caused by lab error. I spent the week being poked and drained of blood until the team of hematologists finally made their announcement: I was now clear to have the surgery in a few days.

THE BACK STORY

Somehow relating this story seems like a bad dream or a nightmare—and it pains me to recall it. During the months leading up to my surgery, my illness journey had already led me through times of hopelessness, depression and even despair. In previous chapters, I shared that Parkinson's causes depression. The earlier bout of depression I faced, however, was light compared to the despair that knocked at my door around the time of the surgery. Maybe it was the vulnerability of writing my story and "putting it all out there." Maybe it was due to a dark secret that had recently come to light. Or maybe it was because I was wrestling with the third phase of Parkinson's and facing serious surgery because of it. (The third phase includes rather severe symptoms such as the inability to walk straight or to stand.) In retrospect, I think it was the combination of all three that left me feeling as if I had been body-slammed to the mat.

There were hidden things in my life—physical and spiritual. A few weeks before the brain surgery, I was hospitalized with a high fever. I was treated for cellulitis, but in the process, a blood clot was discovered in my leg. Had it gone undetected, it could have traveled to my heart during the operation and killed me. God was merciful to reveal its presence beforehand.

Spiritual issues were exposed at the same time—things hidden deep in my heart. In his mercy, God revealed the concealed things, but it felt far from merciful. Through this painful exposure, God was bringing me to repentance and purifying my heart. The surgical procedure involved probing deep into my brain, but first the Holy Spirit had to perform a deep probe into my heart.

After the hidden things were brought to light and addressed, it was as if God said, "Now you can have the operation." The electrodes, foreign objects placed in my brain to block the symptoms of Parkinson's, became a symbol of the way hope would be planted in my soul. Both were painful, but necessary.

Back on the operating table for a second attempt, I was fully conscious. I was aware of the drill's entrance into my skull, heard the saw and felt the pressure of the surgeon cutting into my brain. I said, "Whoa, the sixties are back now! You just blew my mind." The whole operating team laughed. Several assistants said they wanted to be with me the next time because I was so funny. I didn't say it then, but I secretly hoped there wouldn't be a next time!

THE GRACE OF HOPE

James Houston's book *The Transforming Power of Prayer* helped me persevere during this dark period before the surgery. The chapters titled "Deepening Your Friendship with God," "Prayer in Our Woundedness" and "Prayer in Our Fear" spoke to my heart, but none as powerfully as "Prayer in Our Inner Darkness." Houston says, "Encountering darkness in our lives should not drive us *from* prayer, but drive us *to* prayer. Darkness only becomes an obstacle when we fail to see God as the powerful ruler of our lives, able to overcome the evil we face in spite of our own fears and feelings."[1]

I also meditated on this prayer by an early Cistercian monk, Aelred of Rievaulx. He lived in the king's court in Scotland but turned away from privilege to experience a life of prayer in a monastery.

> *Lord, look at my soul's wounds.*
> *Your living and effective eye sees everything.*
> *It pierces like a sword, even to part asunder soul and spirit.*
> *Assuredly, my Lord, you see in my soul the traces of my*
>   *former sin;*
> *My present perils, and also motive and occasions for others . . .*
> *You see these things, Lord, and I would have you see them.*
> *You know well, O searcher of my heart,*
> *That there is nothing in my soul that I would hide from you,*
> *Even had I the power to escape your eyes . . .*
> *Lord, may your good, sweet Spirit descend into my heart,*
> *And fashion there a dwelling for himself,*
> *Cleansing it from all defilement both of flesh and spirit,*

Pouring into it the increment of faith, hope and love,
  Disposing it to penitence and love and gentleness.[2]

The darkness seemed inescapable as I tried to make sense of it all. At this point you are familiar with my journey into grace and may sense that I am usually an optimistic person. The difference between my emotional state when I was first diagnosed and the time of the brain surgery a few years later is a question of hope. In order to experience true hope, I had to walk through complete hopelessness. God doesn't place hope in front of us like a maze, watching to see whether we will find our way to the end. We often become "dashers" against hope—we don't believe, we rebel against hope or we look for hope in the wrong things. In my case, I looked for hope in a "fixed" body and in restored function that would help me keep up with the pack.

I also felt I needed to create my own hope. I hid from my soul's true condition. I submitted to God in some ways, but the Lord wanted to take me deeper. He was dealing with issues that had led to sin, and even though I confessed and turned from my sin and wrongful expectations, those deep-seated habits were replaced with fear, apprehension and doubt that questioned the end result. I wondered whether hope would ever be restored.

I cried with the apostle Paul, "Wretched man that I am! Who will rescue me from this body of death?" (Romans 7:24). In my hopelessness I felt God saying, "My grace is sufficient for you. *Hope in that alone.*"

God's grace brings forth hope; it is birthed into our souls. It's not a wish or a fairy tale. Hope is believing and then trusting in something larger than myself. Hebrews 11:1 says, "Now faith is the assurance of things hoped for, the conviction of things not seen." In the midst of overwhelming difficulties, depression and wondering whether life was worth living, I still held onto the thread of hope that God was faithful, even when I was not. My hope continued to be restored, even in the midst of the painful realities I faced—progressing weakness and illness, strained relationships, and being away from active duty as a priest.

My hope does not depend on any of these things; I'm hopeful because of my friendship with Jesus. Jesus initiates the friendship, as he said, "I do not call you servants any longer . . . but I have called you friends" (John 15:15). Jesus provides an unlimited resource of grace from God—unmerited, undeserved favor in the form of infinite and boundless hope.

My false hopes had to be dashed in order to know true hope. I was trusting in the results of the surgery rather than in the Healer himself. I was attempting to be a good and faithful man, husband and priest, and was trusting in myself and in my ability to do these things well. My hope was misplaced. Hope has a name—and it is *Jesus*. He was pierced, too, and a crown of thorns was thrust upon his head. He despaired in the Garden of Gethsemane, not over his sin but over mine. He understood the darkness. But he overcame it and lived to offer light and grace to all, even me.

HOPE STANDS BEFORE YOU

Hope brings harmony with God through Jesus, a beautiful thing to experience. Again, James Houston puts it this way, "Only a life of awe in God's presence can empower us to live harmoniously, responding to the work of the Holy Spirit within us. Without a sense of awe at God, and harmony with Him, we lose our sense of God's presence with us, for days or even years of our lives."[3] That's the very definition of hopelessness. In Halford Luccock's book *Unfinished Business*, he states that the lack of hope or confidence in the future results in hopelessness in the present.[4]

A scene beside the pool of Bethesda recorded in the Bible illustrates this beautifully (John 5:1-18). A sick man lay beside the pool daily for thirty-eight years. He believed the tradition that, after angels stirred the water, the first person to enter it would be healed. But he could never get there in time to be healed. Imagine how he felt when Jesus stood before him and asked, "Do you want to be made well?" In other words, Jesus was asking, "Do you want to experience life again? Do you want to blossom and flourish once more? Are you willing to acknowledge your sins, which account for your hopelessness and despair? Do you want all the years to mean something—all the times you waited for hope to appear? Then you must listen to my words." At Jesus' command, the man was healed physically and then restored to his family, to society and to himself. Hope stood in front of him—Jesus *was* his only hope, not the waters, not the angels and not someone to lower him into the pool. And Jesus is our hope as well.

Even Jesus had to cling to hope in a desperate time. Hebrews 12:2 tells us that he endured the cross and disregarded its shame because of "the joy that was set before him." The work of redemption—my pardon and yours—was the joy and hope that kept him faithful until the end. This verse also encourages us to "[fix] our eyes on Jesus, the author and perfecter of faith" (NASB). He is our source of hope.

FROM HOPELESS TO HOPEFUL

I heard the story of a missionary from a small Croatian town whose faith exemplifies hope in seemingly hopeless circumstances. Josip Debeljuh was the youngest of three children in a poor family with an alcoholic father and a mentally ill mother. His dad worked a minimum-wage job, and his mother did the best she could to feed her children and show them love. However, he remembers wandering the streets as young as three years old, coming inside only when he was hungry and hoping to find some bread for a meal.

The Debeljuhs were looked down on and teased because of their names. Josip's father was from Kosovo and gave the children names from the Muslim culture instead of the Roman Catholic one in Croatia. (They later changed their names to stop the harassment.) Also, because of his parents' mixed marriage, his mother's family wanted nothing to do with them. They were five poor and despised people living in a small two-bedroom apartment with no shower or bathtub, and sharing a tiny toilet room down the hall. The children basically raised themselves with little or no adult guidance.

Josip was a talented basketball player. One day, he met a man from a Christian college in the United States who offered him a chance to play on their team while getting a college education. Miraculously, his high school principal agreed to give him a diploma even though he dropped out of school in the tenth grade.

Josip says,

Looking back on my life, I would say I was the last candidate to go to college or to graduate, but miracles do happen. At the age of twenty-two, not speaking any English and with only fifty dollars in my pocket (and having borrowed money for the airfare), I was heading to America to study at Belhaven College. A few of the guys were really nice to me and kept inviting me to church. I finally went—the first time I had ever gone to any church. It took awhile, but I eventually surrendered my life to Christ. Before this happened, I would say that basketball saved me and allowed me to escape a desperate situation. Now I know that God gave me the talent and passion for basketball and used it as a tool, not only to bring me to himself, but also to give me value and direction.

I met the love of my life while at Belhaven, and we married after graduation. Through Kelly's dad, I saw what a good husband and father looked like; her parents showed me that it was possible to passionately serve the Lord and have an impact on the community while raising nine children. Now Kelly and I have five children of our own and are serving together as missionaries in my home country of Croatia.

As I reflect on my story, I am amazed at the Lord's grace. I'm sure many people who saw us as children thought, "There is no hope for them." But God had a plan; he brought me out of tremendously difficult circumstances and transformed my life. Often the Lord uses the lowly, the broken and the hopeless to display his glory and power. This is hope—he can use anyone and can bring transformation to the most desperate of lives.

REFLECTION

There are many things that can lead to hopelessness. This is not an exhaustive list, but some symptoms are:

- Being overwhelmed by circumstances, with feelings of being out of control

- Being stuck in a rut emotionally, physically or mentally, and feeling that there is nothing to look forward to

- Being isolated and not being open to suggestions that could possibly bring you out of this place

- A loss of personal vision for your life, with no energy or desire to enter in again and live

- Feeding bad habits like overeating, not taking care of yourself, not getting enough rest or exercise, beating yourself up, over-medicating, etc.

- Giving into despair and anxiety, and believing the lie that there is no hope for getting beyond your circumstances

- Not trusting God as your source of hope, but instead looking to your own resources, which are painfully insufficient

Some ways to counteract this hopelessness:

- Experience God's grace. Visualize bringing your cup to be filled up from his great supply; draw and drink out of the abundance of God's grace that is as unlimited as the ocean.

- Put your hope in God through Jesus Christ rather than in yourself and your efforts to bring about change.

- Become part of a community that can buoy hope, encourage you to trust God and pray for you.

- Focus on gratefulness—there are always things for which to be thankful. Start with something as simple as gratefulness that you woke up this morning, that the sun is shining or for someone's presence in your life.

- Speak words of faith to yourself and others. Declare out loud that your hope is in Christ and cry out to him for deliverance.

- Have a single-minded vision and use Scripture as a guide. An example would be to meditate on Psalm 42:1: "As a deer longs for flowing streams, so my soul longs for you, O God."

Can you remember the last time you felt hopeless? This is not necessarily a bad thing; it can lead you to pursue a deeper relationship with Jesus, who is your hope. It may sounds simplistic, but it can be the source of renewed hope.

Like Josip, hope can lead you to believe for the first time. And like me, in each situation where you find renewed hope, you can choose to believe again. The Bible says, "And hope does not disappoint us, because God's love has been poured into our hearts through the Holy Spirit that has been given to us" (Romans 5:5).

Hope can change when circumstances change. But what happens when circumstances don't change, or when they get worse instead of better? Then our ultimate trust is placed on the hope laid up for us in heaven spoken of in Colossians 1:4-5: "For we have heard of your faith in Christ Jesus and of the love that you have for all the saints, because of the hope laid up for you in heaven." And, as Thomas Brooks said, "Hope can see heaven through the thickest clouds."[5]

May we all have such vision—faith that allows us to set all our hope "on the grace that Jesus Christ will bring you when he is revealed" (1 Peter 1:13). Having biblical hope is not a figment of our imagination but rather a life built and fleshed out through the truths in Scripture.

APPLICATION

Many psalms record emotions of hopelessness yet at the same

time spell out how perfect hope is found in God. Read Psalms 42 and 43 in their entirety, but especially note the refrain:

> Why are you in despair, O my soul?
> And why have you become disturbed within me?
> Hope in God, for I shall again praise Him
> *For the help of His presence.* (Psalm 42:5 NASB, emphasis
>   added)

The writer repeats this in Psalm 43:

> Why are you in despair, O my soul?
> And why are you disturbed within me?
> Hope in God, for I shall again praise Him,
> *The help of my countenance and my God.* (Psalm 43:5 NASB,
>   emphasis added)

When you are hopeful in him, even your countenance changes! And looking up changes our perspective, as another psalm encourages us:

> I lift up my eyes to the hills—
>   from where will my help come?
> My help comes from the LORD,
> who made heaven and earth. (Psalm 121:1-2)

Where are you putting your hope? I encourage you to deepen your friendship with Jesus; he is our hope today and tomorrow.

10

Streams of Grace

The Grace of Living a New Way

🝚

PEOPLE OFTEN TELL ME HOW STRONG I AM and how much courage I display in my walk with Parkinson's. They don't know that, underneath all the bravado, I'm just a little boy who used all his tickets at the fair and has failed to set aside money for the bus ride home.

I'm not sure what's ahead for me, and I find I am increasingly like that frightened boy longing to get home. I relate to the words Twila Paris sang years ago, "They don't know that I go running home when I fall down; they don't know who picks me up when no one is around; I drop my sword and cry for just awhile, 'cause deep inside this armor, the warrior is a child."[1] My future is unclear, and if I allow myself to project, it appears desperately scary. The paralyzing fear quickly spirals out of control when I read one too many websites on the progression of my disease.

Where's my reason for joy? The final victory chapter that speaks of overcoming? In reality, life is just as complicated as it was in the beginning. There is great uncertainty as I prepare to retire and face the last portion of my life. Parkinson's has a growing hold on me. The future includes a second deep brain stimulation to quicken the left side of my brain. The right side has already been done and shown some improvement, but nothing like I had hoped.

I find the more I learn (and write) about grace, the more there is to know. But God is changing me in the process, and hopefully you as well. Peter Marshall once said, "God will never permit any troubles to come upon us unless He has a specific plan by which great blessing can come out of the difficulty."[2] Our difficulties are the platform for God to "show up" in our lives.

I relate to Jacob, with his story of never-ending struggles. The account is a long one, so I'll summarize it here. (You can read the whole story in Genesis 27–32.) Jacob was a man of flawed character—even his name meant "deceiver" or "grabber." God promised him great blessings, but instead of waiting for them, he tried to obtain them on his own. He disguised himself as his brother Esau and came to his blind and ailing father, Isaac. He stole the blessing meant for the eldest son. Because of this, he had to flee from his home when Esau vowed to kill him. He traveled a good distance and worked for his relative Laban. He fell in love with his daughter Rachel and worked to win her hand, but instead of fulfilling his promise, Laban tricked Jacob by giving him her older sister, Leah. The deceiver had been deceived! Jacob worked for fourteen years to obtain his rightful bride, and six more for the flocks he owned.

After serving twenty years—during which his wages were changed ten times—Jacob fled from his abusive father-in-law. With Laban in pursuit of him, his wives and his children, he was then confronted by his older brother, Esau, and his entourage. This is the setting for the scene near the Jabbok River, where Jacob wrestled with an angel of the Lord after falling asleep. He was oppressed coming and going, and greatly troubled in spirit.

God allowed Jacob to go through these difficult experiences for a reason—so that he might come face to face with the man he really was. And when Jacob saw it clearly, the Lord changed his name to Israel, which means "he who strives with God." He emerged from the wrestling match not only with a new name but with a disability that affected him for the rest of his life— walking with a limp. This would be a constant reminder of both the encounter with the living Lord and the call on his life to be God's man. What caused him to wrestle with God? Jacob knew he desperately needed God's blessing to go forward.

The amazing thing about this story is not the tenacity of Jacob but God's grace in using a conniving "grabber" to accomplish his will. God made the same covenant with this flawed man that he made with Abraham and Isaac. He blessed his wives with twelve sons and caused his flocks to flourish. He allowed him to be in the lineage that produced the Messiah.

One commentator writes, "Jacob's wrestling with God at the Jabbok River that dark night reminds us of this truth: Though we may fight God and His will for us, in truth, God is so very good. As believers in Christ, we may well struggle with Him through the loneliness of night, but by daybreak His blessing will come."[3]

And so it is with me. God has revealed more of who I am and caused me to look at the depths of my depravity. In the process, he's shown me more of who he is—a kind, loving, sympathetic, gracious yet holy and righteous Redeemer. I exchanged my unrighteousness for his righteousness through Christ. He's touched not only my thigh but also my whole body, and Parkinson's is my limp. The blessing is to know more of who he is and consider less of myself. Like Jacob, I'm acutely aware that I need his blessing to finish the journey.

In an interview, Billy Graham's grandson Tullian Tchividjian talked about God's amazing grace by saying,

> In those early days [of faith], I was treating the Bible like it was a heaven-sent self-help manual. The fact is, that unless we go to the Bible to see Jesus and his work for us, even our devout Bible reading can become fuel for our own self-improvement plans, the place we go for the help we need to "conquer today's challenges and take control of our lives." What I've learned since those days is that *the Bible is not a record of the blessed good, but rather the blessed*

bad. The Bible is not a witness to the best people making it up to God; it's a witness to God making it down to the worst people. The Bible is one long story of God meeting our rebellion with his salvation; our failure with his favor; our guilt with his grace; our badness with his goodness.[4]

Our story, when all is said and done, will hopefully have one refrain like that of a famous hymn: "Grace, grace, God's grace, grace that will pardon and cleanse within; Grace, grace, God's grace, grace that is greater than all my sin. We who are longing to see his face, will we this moment receive his grace?"[5]

GRACE FOUND NOAH

We're all familiar with the story of Noah and the flood. Because of the corruption of humankind, God was sorry he made humanity and chose to destroy the world (Genesis 6:5-8). By following God's specific instructions, Noah built an ark and escaped with his family, along with two of every animal species on earth.

Genesis 6:8 says, "Noah found favor [grace] in the sight of the LORD." I grew up singing the Negro spiritual that put this same thought to music. But theologian J. A. Motyer says the best way to translate the meaning from the Hebrew is "Grace found Noah." Noah didn't discover or "find" grace; instead, *grace found him.* The difference is significant because the action begins and ends with God being both the initiator and extender of grace.

This is the first time grace is mentioned in the Bible, although the idea had already appeared. At a time when sin was at a high-water mark, grace launched a counteroffensive maneuver. The very meaning of grace implies there is nothing in the man to call it forth or to deserve it. It also reveals a timeless principle: No one ever comes into right relationship with God through his or her own works or righteousness. It is the grace of God, not the graces of Noah, that made the difference!

Encountering God's grace changes a person. In fact, it's the only thing that truly changes a person. We read in Genesis 6:9 of the three effects grace had on Noah. First, he is called a righteous man because of his obedience—grace in "shoe leather." Second, he is called blameless among the people of his time; his private worship became a public witness. And third, he walked with God. The taproot of his faith and the experience of grace led to a godly lifestyle in communion with God.[6]

DIVING INTO GRACE

Recently I had the privilege of visiting a forty-year-old woman in the hospital. Married and the mother of a five-year-old daughter, Dianne was undergoing twenty-four-hour chemotherapy due to the return of cancer. She had also experienced kidney failure and undergone dialysis. Her future seemed bleak, and she greatly missed the normal interaction with her young family as she lay ill in the hospital.

When I walked into the room, she gave me her trademark smile. I asked whether she was hopeful, and she responded, "Not really." I encouraged her to close her eyes and meditate on the ocean, thinking of the water as the grace and love of God. Then I asked her to take her bucket to the shoreline and declare to the ocean, "I'm going to empty you out!" Of course, by the third or fourth try of bailing water, she realized the vast sea made her task hopeless. Then I had her yield to the beauty, fullness and abundance of the water. "Walk in it up to your ankles. Feel it. Now wade in as the waves press your legs more forcefully. As you continue until you are eye level with the water, realize that you are only in a fraction of its depths. Yield yourself completely to the God whose love is as vast as the ocean—throw yourself on his mercy and let his grace carry you."

I asked again whether she was hopeful. She answered, "Yes, my spirit is calm. I am at rest." I kissed her on the cheek with the words, "Be at peace, child."

Having been ministered to in the hospital myself, I realized the value of those words and the power of the interaction. None of us knew that a few days later she would go home to be with the Lord. Those with her at the time said they were amazed at the peacefulness in her death. Grace doesn't run from truth—about yourself, your circumstances or your true condition. It gives you courage to face them all.

THE GRACE OF LIVING A NEW WAY

Hebrews 13:9 says, "It is well for the heart to be strengthened by grace." How are our hearts strengthened by grace? Again, in an interview about his new book, *One Way Love*, Tullian Tchividjian says that only undeserved grace can truly melt and transform the heart. He quotes Charles Spurgeon, who said, "When I thought God was hard, I found it easy to sin; but when I found God so kind, so good, so overflowing with compassion, I beat my breast to think I could ever have rebelled against One who loved me so and sought my good."[7]

Recognizing grace is a learning process. We don't come to this understanding by being smart but by recognizing our need. It is God showing up in our story, revealing more about himself. Like Job, we say, "I had heard of you by the hearing of the ear, but now my eye sees you" (Job 42:5).

My journey has revealed grace through dealing with a disease and walking through the three-step process of acceptance, submission and relinquishment. I have experienced the grace of compassion through Jesus and others around me. I've learned to walk more closely with God through the grace of trust being established in my heart. The grace of community has carried me at times and kept me on the road to faith. I have received the grace of comfort through the nearness of Christ and the love of my family. By necessity I've learned the special ministry of the grace of simplicity, and I've been sustained in dark times by the grace of hope.

Your story may be different from mine, with other aspects of his grace highlighted. Some have told me of their journeys in the grace of perseverance, the grace of humility, the grace of order and the grace of honesty. But these different experiences all come to the same conclusion: "God is faithful; by him you were called into the fellowship of his Son, Jesus Christ our Lord" (1 Corinthians 1:9).

Chapter 12 of Hebrews talks about a "great shaking" that God causes in both the heavens and the earth. This shaking denotes the removal of the things that *can* be shaken so that the things that *cannot* be shaken might remain. I've experienced this shaking and believe the process eventually comes to all true believers in Jesus Christ. Anything that we depend on other than God will be removed, allowing the unshakable things to remain. "Therefore, since we are receiving a kingdom that cannot be shaken, let us give thanks, by which we offer to God an acceptable worship with reverence and awe" (Hebrews 12:28).

The whole book of 1 Peter gives instructions on grace; it was written to Christians suffering persecution to teach them how to stand firm in grace. Each of the five chapters shows a different aspect of grace—grace for salvation (chapter 1), grace for growth (chapter 2), grace for godly living (chapter 3), grace for suffering (chapter 4) and grace for service (chapter 5). The main theme is that suffering and glory go hand in hand. It points to Jesus' example in standing firm in grace: "While being reviled, He did not revile in return; while suffering, He uttered no threats, but *kept entrusting Himself to Him who judges righteously*" (1 Peter 2:23 NASB, emphasis added). Peter's purpose in writing the book was to exhort the believers—and us—that "this is the true grace of God. Stand firm in it!" (1 Peter 5:12 NASB). If Jesus had to continually entrust himself into his Father's grace-filled hands, we must follow his example and do so also.

I don't know what the future holds for me, whether I will be healed of the disease that ravages my body or that one day I will die from its complications. But I know who holds the future—my future—and trust that, like Dianne, he will carry me in his grace and finally bring me home. For, "The one who calls you is faithful, and he will do this" (1 Thessalonians 5:24).

REFLECTION

My story began—and ends—with grace. Sin and discouragement continue to grip my life, but God's grip is stronger. He provides grace each day. I awaken, open the Scriptures and find grace waiting there. I go through emails and find grace in messages others have sent me. I find grace in the letters I receive from many who are praying for me. I have found grace by revealing truth about my life with Parkinson's in this book. And I find grace like the man at the pool who was asked by Jesus, "Do you want to be well?" I look to him as my only hope, the only source of grace.

But even though I think I have found grace, like Noah, *grace has found me.* I wade into its waters and, coming eye level with its fullness, choose to dive into the unfathomable depths of his grace.

What about you? I encourage you to put down your bucket

and stop trying to empty the ocean, or to gain God's favor by your own efforts. It is impossible. Instead, dive into the grace of God and be carried along by the current of his love. Allow yourself to experience the deep, deep love of Jesus.

APPLICATION

In closing, I know of no greater words than those of the hymn "Amazing Grace" to apply to our lives. Although you may have sung these words hundreds of times, I encourage you to read them aloud and apply them to your life. Let them be a means for grace to build your faith and reaffirm the unshakable grace that is ours in Christ.

> *Amazing grace, how sweet the sound,*
> *That saved a wretch like me!*
> *I once was lost, but now am found,*
> *Was blind but now I see.*
>
> *'Twas grace that taught my heart to fear*
> *And grace my fears relieved;*
> *How precious did that grace appear*
> *The hour I first believed!*
>
> *Through many dangers, toils and snares*
> *I have already come;*
> *'Tis grace hath brought me safe thus far,*
> *And grace will lead me home.*

When we've been there ten thousand years,
Bright shining as the sun,
We've no less days to sing God's praise
Than when we first begun.

May the grace of our Lord Jesus Christ be with your spirit. Amen.

ACKNOWLEDGMENTS

MY COAUTHOR, MARJEAN, who has the uncanny ability to take the stumbling words that I offer and create patterns, rhythms and synergy in the written text. For her faithful friendship and the depth of spiritual knowledge and insight she has added to the work. Without her there would be no book.

The community at St. Peter's for their generosity, love and support.

My mentors and friends Richard Foster and Dallas Willard for their consistency in witness, vibrant faith and theological presence in my life.

Cindy Bunch and the entire InterVarsity Press team for their hard work in helping *The Way of Grace* become a reality.

The entire Renovaré team for their friendship throughout the decades.

Susan Tolleson, prinicipal of Propel Book Coaching, for her expert advice and counsel in each stage of development of this book.

Those who allowed me to tell their compelling stories: Mark Ashpole, Andy Russell, Chollet Still, Don Richards and Josip Debeljuh.

Marion, my beloved friend and wife, for her care and commitment.

NOTES

CHAPTER 1: FACING REALITY

[1]Irene Hausherr, *Penthos: The Doctrine of Compunction in the Christian East* (Kalamazoo, MI: Cistercian Publications, 1982), p. 29.

[2]Teresa of Ávila, *The Interior Castle* (Radford, VA: Wilder Publications, 2008), p. 10.

[3]Chris Tiegreen, *The One Year at His Feet Devotional* (Carol Stream, IL: Tyndale House, 2003), July 29, emphasis added.

[4]Max Lucado, *Grace* Participant's Guide (Nashville: Thomas Nelson, 2012), p. 9.

CHAPTER 2: EXPERIENCING THE PRESENCE

[1]St. Ignatius, *The Spiritual Exercises of St. Ignatius*, trans. Anthony Mottola (New York: Doubleday, 1989), pp. 50-52.

CHAPTER 3: GIVING UP

[1]As quoted in Timothy Jones, *Prayer's Apprentice* (Nashville: Thomas Nelson, 2001), p. 211.

[2]Oswald Chambers, *My Utmost for His Highest* (New York: Dodd & Meade, 1985), p. 68.

[3]Elisabeth Elliot, *The Shadow of the Almighty: The Life and Testament of Jim Elliot* (New York: Harper & Brothers, 1956), p. 15.

[4]As quoted in Anne Bogart, *And Then, You Act: Making Art in an Unpredictable World* (New York: Routledge, 2007), p. 97.

CHAPTER 4: STUCK IN AN AIRPORT

[1]As quoted in Mary Penrose, *Refreshing Water from Ancient Wells: The Wisdom of Women Mystics* (Mahway, NJ: Paulist, 2004), p. 36.
[2]Marjean Brooks, © 1978.
[3]As quoted in Terry Glaspey, *25 Keys to Life-Changing Prayer* (Eugene, OR: Harvest House, 2010), p. 140.

CHAPTER 5: GOD IS NOT MAD AT YOU

[1]James A. Sanders, "Hermeneutics," in *The Interpreter's Dictionary of the Bible*, supplementary volume (Nashville: Abingdon, 1976), p. 406.
[2]Frank L. Houghton, *Amy Carmichael of Dohnavur* (Ft. Washington, PA: CLC Publications, 1953). Also, quotes from en.wikipedia.org/wiki/Amy Carmichael.
[3]Amy Carmichael, *The Story of a Fellowship* (Ft. Washington, PA: CLC Publications, 2013), chap. 15.

CHAPTER 6: WOUNDED HEALERS

[1]Joe B. Crowe, "Mountain Brook One of the Wealthiest Communities in US," *The Birmingham News,* December 30, 2008.
[2]For more information on Family Promise, go to www.familypromisebham.org.
[3]Bill White, "Life in Community," *Daymark Counseling Newsletter* (Winter 2013).

CHAPTER 7: A CUP OF COOL WATER

[1]Mother Teresa, *A Simple Path,* ed. Lucinda Vardey (New York: Ballantine Books, 1995), p. xxxii.

[2]Ibid., p. xxxviv.

[3]As quoted in Martin H. Manser, *The Westminster Collection of Christian Quotes* (Louisville, KY: Westminster John Knox, 2001), p. 153.

CHAPTER 8: LIFE IN THE SLOW LANE

[1]Bishop Fenelon, *The Spiritual Letters of Archbishop Fenelon: Letters to Men* (New York: Longmans, Green, and Co., 1914).

[2]Joseph A. Magno, PhD, *The Spiritual Philosophy of the Tao Te Ching* (Chicago: Pendragon Publishing, 2004), p. 115.

[3]Richard Foster, *Celebration of Discipline* (New York: HarperCollins, 1978), p. 79.

[4]Glandion Carney, *Missing Peace* (West Conshohocken, PA: Infinity Publishing, 2013), pp. 158-59.

[5]Augustus M. Toplady, "Rock of Ages," hymn.

[6]Chris Tiegreen, "Simply Focused: Uncluttering the Christian Life." Taken from *indeed magazine* (September/October 2012), pp. 62-64, emphasis added. Used by permission from Walk Through the Bible, www.walkthru.org.

[7]Dr. Kevin Elko, "Growing," free monthly newsletter (April 2013).

CHAPTER 9: POSSIBILITIES

[1]James Houston, *The Transforming Power of Prayer* (Colorado Springs: NavPress, 1996), p. 60, emphasis added.

[2]As quoted in James Houston, *The Prayer: Deepening Your Friendship with God* (Colorado Springs: Cook Communication Ministries, 2007), pp. 61-62.

[3]Houston, *Transforming Power,* p. 61.

[4]As quoted in Jacob Braude, *New Treasury of Stories for Every Speaking and Writing Occasion* (Englewood Cliffs, NJ: Prentice-Hall, 1959), p. 147.

[5]As quoted in Chris Tiegreen, *The One Year at His Feet Devotional* (Carol Steam, IL: Tyndale House, 2003), p. 8.

CHAPTER 10: STREAMS OF GRACE

[1]Twila Paris, "The Warrior Is a Child," *Twila Paris Greatest Hits: Time and Again,* Singspiration Music/ASCAP, 1984.

[2]As quoted in Martin H. Manser, *The Westminster Collection of Christian Quotations* (Louisville, KY: Westminster John Knox, 2001), p. 382.

[3]S. Michael Houdmann, "Question: What is the meaning of Jacob wrestling with God?" www.gotquestions.org/Jacob-wrestling-with-God.html.

[4]Jonathan Merritt, "Billy Graham's Grandson Takes Christians to Task: An Interview with Tullian Tchividjian," *Jonathan Merritt On Faith and Culture* (blog), *Religion News Service,* October 2, 2013, http://jonathanmerritt.religionnews.com/2013/10/02/tullian-tchividjian, emphasis added.

[5]Julia H. Johnston, "Grace Greater Than Our Sin," hymn.

[6]I am deeply indebted to Rev. Ronald Steel of Eastbridge Presbyterian Church in Charleston, South Carolina, for his sermon notes on the subject of grace finding Noah.

[7]Merritt, "Billy Graham's Grandson Takes Christians to Task."

About the Authors

Glandion Carney was formerly a pastor and church planter in the Reformed Church before being ordained as an Anglican priest. He was associate pastor at St. Peter's Anglican Church in Birmingham, Alabama, before retiring from active ministry in November 2013. Glandion was involved in Renovaré for fifteen years in the capacity of spiritual director and board member. He was also chaplain of the Christian Legal Society for twelve years.

Glandion currently lives in Birmingham. He and his wife, Marion, are the parents of four adult children. Glandion enjoys volunteering at the Parkinson's Foundation, where he helps to bring support, encouragement and a listening ear to those going through the ravages of the disease. This is his eighth book.

Marjean Brooks is a writer who lives in Birmingham, Alabama, and attends St. Peter's Anglican Church. She and her husband, Ricky, have six adult children and nine grandchildren.

As a teacher and mentor to hundreds of women during her life, she loves leading in-depth Bible studies and often supplements the teaching with her own writings. Marjean's articles, poetry and devotions have been published in various ministry publications, and she has written a monthly column in *Senior Living* newspaper for many years.

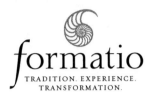

formatio

TRADITION. EXPERIENCE.
TRANSFORMATION.

Formatio books from InterVarsity Press follow the rich tradition of the church in the journey of spiritual formation. These books are not merely about being informed, but about being transformed by Christ and conformed to his image. Formatio stands in InterVarsity Press's evangelical publishing tradition by integrating God's Word with spiritual practice and by prompting readers to move from inward change to outward witness. InterVarsity Press uses the chambered nautilus for Formatio, a symbol of spiritual formation because of its continual spiral journey outward as it moves from its center. We believe that each of us is made with a deep desire to be in God's presence. Formatio books help us to fulfill our deepest desires and to become our true selves in light of God's grace.

What is Renovaré?

Renovaré USA is a nonprofit Christian organization that models, resources, and advocates fullness of life with God experienced, by grace, through the spiritual practices of Jesus and of the historical Church. We imagine a world in which people's lives flourish as they increasingly become like Jesus.

Through personal relationships, conferences and retreats, written and web-based resources, church consultations, and other means, Renovaré USA pursues these core ideas:

- *Life with God* - The aim of God in history is the creation of an all-inclusive community of loving persons with God himself at the center of this community as its prime Sustainer and most glorious Inhabitant.

- *The Availability of God's Kingdom* - Salvation is life in the kingdom of God through Jesus Christ. We can experience genuine, substantive life in this kingdom, beginning now and continuing through all eternity.

- *The Necessity of Grace* - We are utterly dependent upon Jesus Christ, our ever-living Savior, Teacher, Lord, and Friend for genuine spiritual transformation.

- *The Means of Grace* - Amongst the variety of ways God has given for us to be open to his transforming grace, we recognize the crucial importance of intentional spiritual practices and disciplines (such as prayer, service, or fasting).

- *A Balanced Vision of Life in Christ* - We seek to embrace the abundant life of Jesus in all its fullness: contemplative, holiness, charismatic, social justice, evangelical, and incarnational.

- *A Practical Strategy for Spiritual Formation* - Spiritual friendship is an essential part of our growth in Christlikeness. We encourage the creation of Spiritual Formation Groups as a solid foundation for mutual support and nurture.

- *The Centrality of Scripture* - We immerse ourselves in the Bible: it is the great revelation of God's purposes in history, a sure guide for growth into Christlikeness, and an ever rich resource for our spiritual formation.

- *The Value of the Christian Tradition* - We are engaged in the historical "Great Conversation" on spiritual formation developed from Scripture by the Church's classical spiritual writings.

Christian in commitment, ecumenical in breadth, and international in scope, Renovaré USA helps us in becoming like Jesus. The Renovaré Covenant succinctly communicates our hope for all those who look to him for life:

> In utter dependence upon Jesus Christ as my ever-living
> Savior, Teacher, Lord, and Friend,
> I will seek continual renewal through:
> • spiritual exercises • spiritual gifts • acts of service

RENOVARÉ

Renovaré USA
8 Inverness Drive East, Suite 102 • Englewood, CO, 80112 USA • 303-792-0152
www.renovare.us